Advance Praise for *Surviving the Cancer System:*

"Dr. Fesen shines a spotlight on the cancer system from both sides of the stethoscope. His honest and thorough assessment allows cancer patients to better understand the importance of being a participant in their own care. His straightforward 'tell it like it is' approach provides the tools needed to relinquish the role of 'cancer victim' and empowers the patient to successfully navigate their own cancer journey. In 25 years of working with cancer patients, I have not seen a more comprehensive and helpful overview of this topic, and it is a 'must-read' for anyone touched by cancer!"

—Diana Thomi, RN, BS, Executive Director,
Victory in the Valley, Inc.

"Dr. Fesen has drawn back the curtain and exposed the inner workings of the cancer system—all of the barriers that cancer patients face in their efforts to fight a terrible disease. But this book will bring patients one giant step closer in a journey that, now more than ever, has more hope than despair."

—Virginia Stark-Vance, MD, coauthor,
100 Questions and Answers About Brain Tumors

"Mark, thank you. Cancer is indeed a systemic disease, and you give us both personal and objective insights into the multiple human, social, economic, and medical aspects of cancer. [This] book meets the challenge of containing a wealth of practical information while being remarkably easy to read. It covers so many aspects of cancers that all of us, patients, family members, physicians, and caregivers, will find it a long-lasting reference. It is an honest and often moving account of cancer patients and of your experiences. I recommend this book to cancer patients, libraries, and health professionals."

—Dr. Yves Pommier, National Cancer Institute Lab Director

". . . a must-have for all cancer patients."

—M. L. Dubay, nine-year cancer survivor and coauthor,
100 Questions and Answers About Brain Tumors

D1110394

"A carefully considered, detailed examination of the various aspects of the journey the new cancer patient will experience."

—Rue McClanahan, cancer survivor and actress

"I was diagnosed with cancer at the age of 33. I had never been sick and my daughter was a month old. I was scared to death. I was blessed to have Dr. Fesen as my oncologist. I wish I had had this book!"

—Kevin O'Connor, Deputy District Attorney, Wichita, Kansas

"Today, entering the complex world of healthcare delivery with the diagnosis of a life-threatening illness is a fearful experience for the patients we serve through Patient Advocate Foundation. They are often battling diagnosis of disease, financial hurdles with lost employment, and out-of-pocket costs while seeking to assure themselves and their loved ones that they are making the best treatment decisions. Dr. Fesen's book is a primer in patient empowerment offering concrete patient stories that capture the essence of the patients' struggles and their successes. The book compels you to keep reading and to find solutions as noted in Chapter 7, "Insurance Angles: Making the System Work for You." His approach to simplifying complex information encourages readers to find solutions for themselves and assures them they are not alone in the journey."

—Nancy Davenport-Ennis, CEO, Patient Advocate Foundation

Surviving the Cancer System

An Empowering Guide to Taking Control of Your Care

Mark R. Fesen, MD, FACP

AMACOM

American Management Association
New York • Atlanta • Brussels • Chicago • Mexico City
San Francisco • Shanghai • Tokyo • Toronto • Washington, D.C.

This publication is designed to provide accurate and authoritative information in regard to the
subject matter covered. It is sold with the understanding that the publisher is not engaged in
rendering legal, accounting, or other professional service. If legal advice or other expert assistance is required, the services of a competent professional person should be sought.

Various names used by companies to distinguish their software and other products can be claimed
as trademarks. AMACOM uses such names throughout this book for editorial purposes only, with
no intention of trademark violation. Individual companies should be contacted for complete information regarding trademarks and registration.

The advice concerning drug treatment options is believed to be accurate. However, neither the
authors nor the publisher can accept legal responsibility for possible errors in or adverse consequences from the use of these drugs. It is the responsibility of practitioners to check the pack-
aging information as well as to confirm information with the manufacturer.

The diagnosis, selection, and administration of cancer treatment is a highly complex and ever-
evolving process that must be tailored to the specific circumstances and needs of each patient.
The discussion in this book is not intended to be relied upon as a substitute for such specifically
tailored medical advice and treatment.

Library of Congress Cataloging-in-Publication Data

Fesen, Mark R.
    Surviving the cancer system : an empowering guide to taking control of
your care / Mark R. Fesen.
        p. cm.
    Includes index.
    ISBN-13: 978-0-8144-1356-2 (pbk.)
    ISBN-10: 0-8144-1356-0 (pbk.)
    1. Cancer—Popular works.   2. Self-care, Health.   I. Title.
RC263.F46 2009
616.99′4—dc22   2009009838

Printing number

10 9 8 7 6 5 4 3 2

To my dad, Robert Fesen, the finest man I've ever known. He lived his life with humility, honesty, and integrity. He also taught me that throughout life I would find many who are better than I and that I should learn from them. This attitude has helped me gain much from patients, families, and coworkers. One of his favorite quotes was from Rudyard Kipling and seems uniquely appropriate to the attitude and work of an oncologist:

". . . By the livin' Gawd that made you,
You're a better man than I am, Gunga Din!"

Contents

Author's Note   ix

Acknowledgments   xi

1   Surviving the System
You're Fighting More Than an Illness   1

2   The Sudden Cancer Panic Syndrome
Don't Pay the High Price of Panic   8

3   Your Most Important Relationship
How Your Oncologist Measures Up   16

4   Cooperation and Consensus
Bonding with Your Oncology Team   29

5   Understanding Cancer
It's Not Just One Disease   39

6   Major Cancer Centers
What Every Patient Should Know   48

7   Insurance Angles
Making the System Work for You   70

8 Chemotherapy, Radiation, Surgery
Innovations, Promises, and Pitfalls 88

9 The Pharmaceutical Industry
Friend or Foe? 105

10 Making Your Own Luck
Tested Ways to Improve Survival Chances 119

11 Back to Your Life
When to Say "Yes" to Travel, Work, Exercise, and Sex 134

12 Supportive Care Insights
How to Better Tolerate Treatment 145

13 Clinical Wisdom
How I Might Do It 156

14 Lymphomas, Myeloma, Leukemias, and Other Blood Cancers
Frequently Overlooked Problems 196

15 The Hospice Dilemma
Why It's Not Always the Answer 212

16 Hands-On Practical Help and Public Policy Advocacy
How You Can Make a Difference for Cancer Patients 224

Appendix 50 Questions and Answers
What My Patients Ask 243

Resources 254

Index 265

About the Author 274

Author's Note

Cancer is not only a disease. It is a highly sophisticated, multifaceted, multibillion dollar system. The sooner you learn how to navigate this system, the more coordinated and effective your care will be.

I wrote this book because I wanted to make a difference. As an oncologist and patient advocate, I was grateful for my practice and moved by the fact that so many of my patients felt bonded to me. They experienced what I wish for all cancer patients—a personal bond with an oncologist who is able to provide the latest coordinated therapies close to home and in a caring environment.

It is my hope this book can provide that for you and your loved ones.

Acknowledgments

This work has been an amalgam of ideas and insights from many people. I am merely the observer and recorder. Many insights are those common within the oncology world where I work.

To my family: Thank you, Mary, my dedicated wife, for putting up with the long hours this manuscript took to compile. You've been wonderful and patient. To Zach, Joy, and Rachael, my children, thanks for being you. Lilly and Moses also contributed their own parts.

To my patients: As you suffer, triumph, and persist, I have learned much from each of you. My intention is always to comfort. It is an honor to have the opportunity to serve.

Cancer changes people and often brings out much of the best in those forced to endure it. This visible change in your persona is a hard won reward that others rarely find. Above all, I appreciate the gritty determination that I have seen in so many. I hope that others will be inspired by your example, as I was once inspired by Tracy, a special and courageous young woman.

To the caring families: Through this trying time in your life, you have taught endurance, patience, and fortitude. I marvel at your dedication to others.

To my coworkers: I appreciate your being willing to work and learn alongside me. Lori Williams is the best physician's assistant in the world.

Her attention to details and her clinical acumen are second to none. The nurses of the Hutchinson Clinic Oncology Department are an inspired group. Mary Ellen, Rosalie, Beulah, Alice, Jennifer, Barb, Linda and all of the others all bring love to their duties. My office staff, including Michele and Dawn, bring a lighthearted nature that calms and reassures in a way I can't. Darlene is uniquely able to triage and communicate with even the most difficult-to-find consultants. Emily, Deb, Delori, and Shelly are great at helping while we see patients. The Promise Regional Medical Center nursing staff is excellent.

To Barb: Thanks for being my teacher, coworker, confessor, and friend. I owe more to you than I can ever repay. You're the best, and you know it. Now the world does too.

To Bob Sourk: Without your wisdom and friendship, Hutchinson would be a much different place. To Murray Holcomb; thanks for all you've taught me. To Steve Braun; thanks for the wonderful attention and care to our patients. To Fadi Estephan; thanks for the excellent care and discussions—you've been a great partner. To my physician partners at the Hutchinson Clinic: thanks for all of your support. To all of the physicians and others who have referred patients to our practice: Thanks for your confidence in me and our team. To Virginia Stark-Vance: I appreciate your inspiration and fearlessness. You've been a good friend. To Tito Fojo, Kevin O'Connor, and Jack Wortman: thanks for reviewing the manuscript in progress. To Robin Durrett, Dan Witt and Nathan and Cameron Knackstedt you guys are great friends and great physicians.

To Bonnie Hearn Hill: WOW!!!!! You once said that I'm only allowed five exclamation points per lifetime. They all are given to you because of the tremendous work you've done. You've been an outstanding help and inspiration. Your help has certainly greatly exceeded my expectations, and this effort is better because of you. I valued our long discussions. Thanks also to Bonnie's assistant, Brooke.

I would also like to acknowledge the dedication and assistance of my agent, June Clark, at FinePrint Literary Agency, Hazel Dixon-Cooper for her early input, Maria Kicklighter, organization wizard, Bob Shuman, my editor at AMACOM. I gratefully appreciate the dedication, expertise, and industriousness of Barbara Chernow. I woud also like to recognize the assistance of Alice Northover, Paula Levine, Jenny Wesselmann Schwartz, Erika Spelman, and Andy Ambraziejus at AMACOM.

Finally, I would like to acknowledge the person who has molded and guided me from birth. This person has devoted her life to the very challenging job of raising four sons. Firsthand, at her apron, I learned about common decencies of caring for others, being polite, and apologizing when wrong. She didn't need to discuss or profess catholic social justice concerns; she lived them. Helping others was second nature to her, as she demonstrated by caring for my bedridden father on a daily basis for the last five years of his life. My mom, Rosemary Fesen, has always been my best teacher.

Chapter 1

Surviving the System
You're Fighting More Than an Illness

Her name is Kelly and, in 1995, she was diagnosed with stage IV lung cancer. What?, you ask. Shouldn't an advanced lung-cancer patient be dead by now?

Apparently not, because as I write this, she planning a trip to France. I use her as an example, not just because she is one of the people many would label "lucky," but because of the type of patient she is—the type of patient I hope you would be if you were in her place.

When Kelly was diagnosed, she quit smoking. She established positive relationships with her doctors, and she got the most mileage she could out of the available therapy. As drugs and treatments changed, she moved to different therapies. In short, she gave herself the chance to be lucky.

She could have sat in a bar and smoked herself to death. But she—and you—will never find out if you are one of the patients with a long-term chance unless you try. If you sit at the bar and smoke and die, you won't be alive in six months when a new and promising drug comes out.

In this book, you will learn that the type of care you receive has little to do with the type of cancer you have and much to do with the type of patient you are. That doesn't mean that you have to be rich or brilliant or contribute large amounts of money to the local clinic. You just have to be prepared, have to have a cooperative attitude, and not look like a lawsuit waiting to happen.

If the doctor is concerned that you or your family members are confrontational or litigious, he may say, "Here are your treatment choices," without taking the risk of influencing you one way or the other.

You, on the other hand, should want to develop a relationship with your doctor that makes her feel comfortable in the role of guide. This book will show you how to accomplish that goal. It is intended as your road map to some new and sometimes frightening territory.

The vast majority of patients think that cancer is one disease that can just flow over your body and take your life. Not so. When lung cancer spreads to your brain, it's not a brain tumor; it's still lung cancer.

Once you have cancer, you become part of a system. Think of it as a musical production in which you are at the mercy of an orchestra of highly skilled performers who must work singularly but in harmony while led by the oncologist conductor. You might prefer to think of it as an athletic event, a basketball game, maybe, with your oncologist as coach. Regardless of the comparison you prefer, you are now part of a system. This system can work for you or against you. There may be harmony or discord. The right conductor-coach-oncologist can determine that, and so can you. This book will help you become receptive to the advice of your conductor/coach, as well as help you choose the right one for you.

Many encyclopedic books on the market explain cancer in great detail. Although we will look at the basics here, this book is your guide to surviving the cancer-care system. If you're tired of bouncing from one doctor and one opinion to another, if you're totally confused and unsure as to where you should turn, you will find answers here. They may not be always pretty or politically correct, but they are as honest as if you were sitting here in front of me asking your questions in person. I hope that's how you'll feel as you read this book.

I want to show you how the system works and where you fit into the great play or ballgame that is cancer. We'll discuss creative ways to get insurance once you have cancer and weigh the differences between staying in your own town or traveling to a major cancer center. We'll also look at the Medicare D plans, explore the hospice system, and define what's really meant when doctors or family members bring up "quality of life" issues. I'll also share with you my Fesen Will-to-Live Scale and offer advice that has helped many of my patients navigate the cancer system.

You have to climb a lot of mountains to see the view. I'm in the unusual position of seeing between 30 and 50 patients with different types of cancer five days a week. I've been doing this for fifteen years.

In addition to my number of years as a practitioner and the number of patients I've seen, this book is based on my experience. Just as important, maybe even more important, it's based on my level of training. That training enables me to work hands on with not just breast cancer patients or lung cancer patients, but patients with hundreds of different types of cancer. It's just me, not me and a fellow, not me and a committee.

Years of experience have shown that cancer care is often poorly organized and frequently chaotic. Insured or not, rich or poor, the current system focuses on care for which a provider can be reimbursed or for which a researcher can add a number to a study. Many patients aren't receiving the coordinated comprehensive care they deserve. Care received after a study is completed or a procedure is finished is often limited at best.

Innumerable calls from friends, friends of friends, relatives, and distant acquaintances have shown me that people are looking for direction. People are looking for someone to give them truthful information. Even if the news is bad, they want honesty. *What is this disease that I have and where should I turn? Whom do I trust? If a famous actor had the same pancreatic cancer and he only took the herbal treatment, should I do so also? If a research fellow at a major cancer center told me that there is nothing more that can be done, should I give up?*

A young man in his forties, a friend of my brother's from a Chicago suburb with several small children, called desperate to understand his very deadly small cell lung cancer. Despite several months of oncology care, he still had not internalized a good understanding of his situation. My goal is to direct him to good local care, but the least that I want to do is give him something that he is searching for—the gift of an understanding of where he stands now. Honesty. *Am I curable? Will I die of this soon?*

A family friend in New Jersey has prostate cancer. He's in his seventies and has been to both his local urologist and to the "expert" at the major cancer center. After he leaves the appointment at the center, he's just as confused as he was when he was diagnosed. *Am I treatable? How long will I live? Who will help me? What doctor do I see who will care for me during this illness?* These are the people for whom this book is intended. I hope that that they and others will be able to use the information here to receive the care they deserve.

Multiple reasons exist for receiving less than perfect care. Misunderstandings about cancer abound. Volunteer advice from the general public often encourages decisions that rely on mythology about cancer. Some providers deliberately exploit confusion about the nature of standard versus alternative therapy. Some patients don't even attempt to receive care fearing that exorbitant costs will bankrupt their survivors. Still others abandon care because of a combination of depression and poor understanding about the benefits of treatment. Horrible legends about the feared short- and long-term side effects of radiation therapy and chemotherapy have paralyzed others who are unable to commit to a decision. Simple medications useful to treat common side effects aren't used when they need to be. Information about new innovations is provided piecemeal to the general public, giving all of us a confusing picture about where the art and possibilities of oncology now stand.

Jack: Drugs, Yes, Chemotherapy, No

At 87, Jack had been suffering from newly diagnosed diabetes, as well as blood clots in his legs that wouldn't resolve. He'd also lost 40 pounds by the time he was referred. He had been hospitalized numerous times over the several months prior to his diagnosis for treatment of his blood clots and diabetes. Eventually a CAT scan was done; it showed a mass in his pancreas, worrisome for pancreatic cancer. The primary care physician asked for an oncology consultation to help make plans for further evaluation and to review treatment options. The patient's son was aware that pancreatic cancer was a likely diagnosis. The doctor reviewed all of the available treatment options, including surgery, radiation, and chemotherapy. At his age of 87, physicians and family all quickly came to a consensus that surgery would be considered only as a last resort. A needle biopsy, they hoped, would be the safest way to diagnose the pancreatic cancer. As the discussion continued, the doctors explained to him and his family that there were nonsurgical means of treatment, including chemotherapy and radiation. The doctors explained that if the biopsy found pancreatic cancer, they would then ask him to consider the standard IV treatment drug, Gemzar (gemcitabine). After listening to the risks and benefits, the patient said the treatment sounded reasonable to him. The side effects were modest and spared any loss of hair. The doctors felt that his quality of life would be better if his cancer and its symptoms could be treated: his family was most concerned about his quality of life. He, his family, and his physicians all agreed that a biopsy would be done and Gemzar, a type of chemotherapy for pancreatic cancer, would be the initial option for treatment.

After the plan was made, Jack and his family were pleased and commented that they were glad that he wouldn't need any *chemotherapy*. After the doctors reexplained to them that Gemzar was a cancer drug and a type of chemotherapy, they were confused. Jack, his family, and all of their friends knew that everyone who received chemotherapy lost their hair, lost weight, and had difficulty controlling vomiting. Jack's children were adamant that they didn't want that for their dad. The doctors had another lengthy discussion with them, explaining that hundreds of different types of medications are included in the family of drugs known as chemotherapy. Each of these drugs has different side effects to treat the many different types of cancer. Patients treated with Gemzar frequently improve their quality of life, the doctor said. After this lengthy discussion, the patient and family agreed to the biopsy and the initiation of treatment.

Practicing in rural central Kansas has provided me with an unusual perch from which to view the cancer world. Pharmaceutical companies provide expert physicians who are willing to travel to this small community to educate us. Their off-the record comments confirm our suspicions about how fortunate the patients in our community are when they are able to receive comprehensive care at home. Still other physicians marvel at the collegial relationships and conversations with government officials that are possible in a smaller community. The stoic, tolerant people in this state have blessed me with the opportunity to serve them and their families for fifteen years. I have learned greatly from this experience. Their stories and others can educate and inspire you and your family.

Experience is a great teacher. Seeing thousands of patients a year suffering from hundreds of different types of cancers has given me a bit of wisdom to share. Many oncologists have been called to serve the thousands suffering from cancer each year. Some work tirelessly treating patients within clinical trials programs that advance our cancer knowledge for the benefit of all of us. However, few understand how much work desperately needs to be done to educate the general public about this disease. And not all are willing to take the time and make the effort to change this.

Many want to help, try to help, and are helping. Others are frustrated because their help isn't fruitful. Well-intentioned federal officials want to be able to approve new drugs but need to abide by strict federal regulations. Physicians try to help their patients by advocating with insurers and bureaucrats. Researchers hope that their trials will enhance our knowledge but know that each study improves our understanding only a little and are frustrated when the FDA does not approve a drug. Alternative providers bravely think outside the box in desperate hopes. Family members seek out any and all help they are able to find from any source. They look up information on the Internet, ask neighbors, and try home remedies. But many treatments still fail you, the patient.

The safety of having a trusting relationship with an oncologist and primary care provider can make all the difference in the world to an ill patient. When this type of relationship replaces a bureaucratic, authoritarian, and scheduled-appointments-only type of relationship, patients are less intimidated and feel comfortable asking the *dumb questions* early that save lives. You, the patient, need to be the priority, not the physician. Your quality of life is what counts. To help relieve suffering at this time of your life, you are the center of the universe.

Surviving the Cancer System will provide practical advice about how to best navigate this system. Even though the essential parts of the narratives are real, the stories are changed to protect patient privacy. Physicians and scientists are trained to understand how to treat cancer based on data in research studies, but describing the latest research study meta-analysis is overwhelming to many. Although clinical trials are essential to expand our knowledge, most of us learn best through anecdotes. Hearing a favorable story about a recommended type of treatment will do much to help most people understand it. Accounts such as those in this book are needed to translate research findings to everyday experiences that patients understand.

I wrote this book because maybe someone, somewhere—a cancer patient or family member—or even a whole lot of "someones" who will never show up in my clinic will pick it up. And maybe that person or those people will find help, even hope, within these pages. That is my belief. It is my heartfelt goal.

EMPOWER YOURSELF

Your behavior and attitude make a huge difference. The system isn't going to treat everyone the same. Knowing how the cancer system works can save your life.

WHAT'S NEXT

A cancer diagnosis generates a single response: fear. Chapter 2 will show you how to keep that fear from destroying your health, your chances to survive, and your life.

Chapter 2

The Sudden Cancer Panic Syndrome
Don't Pay the High Price of Panic

Newly diagnosed patients often arrive in my office in a full-blown panic. At times all they know is that they have cancer and need to quickly see the oncologist. Some are even notified over the phone by a nurse. Most expect to die. Soon. The diagnosing physician, fearing that he may say the wrong thing to an already distraught patient, reasonably decides to have the oncologist quarterback the advice and begin to organize some plans. Many patients are so upset they are unable to remember simple facts about their own lives or recent symptoms. Others cry. All need reassurance, sympathy, and a plan.

New patients are given fistfuls of complex educational material and a packed schedule of tests, clinic visits, and procedures. But it is the reassurance of compassion that calms those who have been found to have cancer. Those who were diagnosed at surgery frequently need to convalesce before beginning chemotherapy. Although doctors don't always see the need for an immediate consult with the oncologist, patients need education. They need hope, they need a plan, and they need it now, not two weeks or a month from now.

Often, when patients look back months later, they hardly remember any information from that first visit. What they do remember are the attitude, the promise, and the hope. The oncologist should leave you with the promise that he will do his best to care for you. Scheduling your first visit as soon as possible will help avoid further apprehension. If you undergo several weeks of bad assumptions, limitless advice from well-intentioned friends, and hollow promises from providers of questionable therapies, you may arrive bewildered and confused.

Patients who are panicked rarely make wise decisions. Physicians, nurses, family members, and others grow frustrated with them because of this. Providers frequently use leading questions to facilitate a decision. "You don't really want to have an operation, do you?" or "I wouldn't want to be placed on a ventilator, would you?" These types of questions fail to get to the issue of what you, the patient, want. Patients who are imprisoned by their panic leave themselves vulnerable to these leading questions and the skewed and rash decisions that may result. By addressing your panic and anxiety, you will be able to process information and make better decisions.

It is common to listen to neighborhood coffee shop advice from people whom you have learned to trust. Patients solicit information from girlfriends, ministers, relatives, teachers, nurse friends, and anyone who will give an opinion. Advice overload often ensues, and the patient is left dazed and confused about where to turn.

Patients take advice from those with whom they have already developed a trusting relationship. Questionable recommendations from a good friend is trusted far more than advice from a senior medical expert in the field. Thoughts from someone trained to spin pseudoscience with warm fuzzy emotional overtones is taken to heart. When the patient finally arrives to listen to the oncologist's opinion, he often discounts the information because at times little or no effort is made by either side to first solidify the relationship and build a foundation of trust.

The neighbor has a history of such trust. The purveyor of dubious medicine has been trained about the importance of building such a relationship. The oncologist, however, rarely appreciates the need to spend time on such matters. His philosophy may well be a condescending one: *Why wouldn't anyone take my word as gospel?* Because of their status, many physicians expect patients to naturally appreciate the wisdom they are imparting to them.

Not appreciating the need to first build a trusting relationship is one of the biggest errors in medicine today. When patients begin to solicit advice regarding treatment options, this trust becomes profoundly important. It's your life. You want to:

- Understand your situation.
- Calmly review all of your options.
- Discuss the advice with your loved ones.
- Then decide for yourself.

THE REALITY OF PHYSICIAN BIAS

Doctors are human. Your physician has had years of training and experience in diagnosing and treating cancer. He has seen many similar patients. He is not in a panic. The physician's stated goals are to evaluate, educate, and help treat. But his one-sided experience may have created a hidden agenda unknown even to him. That agenda is a bias. It may be the surgeon who enjoys the challenge of surgery and wants to cut; the medical oncologist who believes his chemotherapy protocol is best; the radiation oncologist, who is most comfortable with his own treatments and suggests radiation; or the hospice physician, who in his compassion wants to stop treatment and comfort you. Before you can determine the best route for treating your condition, you need to quickly accept the condition you have. Once you've done that, you're better able to recognize these biases and make decisions based on what is right for you.

THE REALITY OF PATIENT BIAS

You may find it difficult to keep an open mind at this time. Patients frequently refuse modern and tolerable therapy because of painful memories of family members who suffered through antiquated treatments. Although such therapies may share only a name—chemotherapy, for instance, they may be one and the same to the patient. A patient may refuse radiation treatment to her breast because of memories of Aunt Sally's radiation burns to her abdomen fifteen years ago. Another patient may refuse chemotherapy without realizing that today's drugs are more targeted, tolerable, and effective than the ones used in the past.

You need to put your bias aside. Keep an open mind to the usefulness of modern treatments.

Louis: Patient Prejudice Limits Therapy Options

Louis is a 74-year-old retired builder who developed a cancer of the mouth area. The lesions rapidly worsened and grew to become an ulcer outside the skin. Due to the dramatic worsening of the mass, his family physician quickly referred him to a major cancer center. They documented that the patient was given the choice of several types of treatment, including surgery, radiation alone, chemotherapy and radiation, or comforting measures. The patient met with only the surgeon and remembers only the surgery recommendations. Louis was not notified of the recommendations of the tumor board, which met the evening before his surgery. Although he was obviously told about the other types of treatment available, the patient only internalized the surgery option. To him, cutting out the cancer was the only option, even before he talked to any surgeon.

His surgery was a success in that the tumor was completely excised and has not recurred. In terms of cosmetic and functional aspects, however, it was a failure. Constant drooling, poor swallowing and aspiration were far worse than Louis expected. And they were irreversible. Other options also have irreversible consequences and are not perfect, but Louis really never considered them.

ACCEPTING YOUR DIAGNOSIS

Get a copy of your pathology report. It's a detailed report describing the microscopic findings of your biopsy. It tells your physicians about the nature of the cancer. Is it aggressive or slow changing? Was it completely removed or is some remaining at the edge? All of this information is included in this important report. Does the document hedge or waffle? Has the pathologist shown the material to another pathologist? To an expert?

Keep your pathology report with you. Read it. Become familiar with it. Post it on the refrigerator as a challenge. Ask questions about the details.

Look up the information in it. It is very important. The first step to accepting the diagnosis of cancer is in understanding what it is you have.

At times, patients feel reassured by having a second pathology department review the material. This is commonly done and is a routine request. Patients can ask for a second opinion in a number of circumstances. Get one if there is any ambivalence in the diagnosis. If the first pathologist report hedges, get a second opinion. If you have decided on a conservative course of treatment, if you have decided against receiving another treatment, get a second opinion, especially if you are young. If the diagnosis seems particularly unexpected or unusual for your age or situation, get another point of view. For example, an elderly male patient of mine was diagnosed with testicular cancer at an unusually old age. In fact, the university had his testicular cancer specimen kept at a center specializing in these tumors, as his was one of the oldest such cancers on record. The second opinion was reassuring to both the patient and me. We knew the diagnosis was correct, and he could move on to his treatment with confidence.

Discussing your cancer diagnosis with friends is healthy. You don't have to ask their opinions. Instead, explain what you've learned. It is by informing others that we learn and internalize best. This helps everyone be more open about the diagnosis of cancer.

ACCEPTANCE, NOT DENIAL

The diagnosis of cancer carries with it such a dread that many patients simply can't accept it. Stories of profound denial abound. One patient, a nurse, ultimately came to the office with a large, draining breast cancer covered up by gauze and perfume. Another, a young man in his twenties, just continued shaving off the melanoma, a fatal type of skin cancer, growing near his sideburns. Denial is a very strong drive and emotion. When the information is this bad, our minds simply won't let it in. They turn elsewhere to more pleasant thoughts of ballgames, work, or friends. Still other patients have never taken the time to learn about cancer and arrive completely uninformed.

Some arrive with an inexhaustible number of excuses as to why the worsening cough is just a smoker's hack. Or why the back pain is just an old work injury and not cancer in the spine. One man had to literally crawl out to his car. His back pain was that bad. Some patients object to gentle encouragement to address the issue. Thus, family members also gradually learn to ignore the problem and become excellent enablers. People eventually adapt to lower and lower levels of functioning. Rather than seeing a lung doctor, a patient in denial will choose to avoid family gatherings where he'd be expected to be active.

Denial is too costly. It can rob you of time. And time represents hope and success. Finding a cancer several months earlier in many cases could represent a significant improvement in chances for cure. Often families help patients through this denial by insisting the patient seek attention. Commonly, an elderly patient's child will bring in Dad during a holiday visit. Not until this time, will the patient's true degree of decline become evident.

Remember: Early cancer is hard to detect, but easy to treat. Advanced cancer is easy to detect, but hard to treat. Denial gives cancer the advantage to become advanced.

THE FIRST VISIT

At first visits, some patients bring as many nearby family members as they can muster. Others come with only a child or spouse. At times, elderly women will bring a friend. Men often arrive alone to the first oncologist visit. It is helpful to have two sets of ears listening to the physician's advice. When the group becomes unwieldy, with more than four people, it becomes challenging for the physician to communicate effectively. Many anxious patients take notes to better remember the advice. It is preferable to have a companion do this so you can better focus on what is being explained. Patients who are trying to write down every word often lose the big picture. Rarely will oncologists have the patience to wait for anyone to write the answers to a long litany of questions. Often one visit is not enough to understand and explain a situation. You and your oncologist will probably both need several visits to completely understand the situation.

Patients who are calmer and less panicked also appear more mature to the oncologist. Physicians are less apt to worry about liability concerns with them. Apprehensive and disturbed patients concern physicians. In most situations, a wide latitude of treatment options are appropriate. The most defensible choices are given to those patients seen as a liability risk. Many subtle clues and nuances happen in the exam room to give the oncologist an idea of how conservative or aggressive his or her advice should be.

ATTITUDE

Attitude greatly affects the chances of success treatment. Enthusiastic patients willing to attack their disease generate an infectious spirit. Physicians and staff enjoy the energy they bring to the office. Such people stay involved. Looking forward to trips, anniversaries, and family events keeps the patient involved in the game of life. When a patient discovers there might be only a limited amount of time remaining, how he or she fills the day becomes important. Despite fatigue, many patients still live life to the fullest.

Depression is a common reaction to a diagnosis of cancer that clouds the ability to make decisions. All of the plans and expectations that you had for the future have changed overnight. When you're depressed, you see all of the reasons to give up. With so many negative outcomes possible, the depressed outlook takes over, and progress grinds to a halt. All options seem futile. Some depressed patients seem to view cancer as a welcome and socially acceptable version of passive suicide. They may appear to think: *If I give up and refuse treatment, I will gain attention as well as get what I've been too insecure to do myself.* It can be necessary to defer cancer therapy several weeks until the depression is treated.

Sometimes family members have bravely helped to re-create a will to live in the patient. Some have gone to great lengths to show their love and compassion.

Jean: Effective Therapy Is Not Always Enough

Stan was a young father with three grade school children. His wife Jean prided herself on her looks. She exercised daily, wore fashionable clothes, and enjoyed going out with her women friends. When her cancer spread five years later, Jean found the cosmetic changes associated with developing metastatic breast cancer especially painful. Hair loss, weight gain, and skin changes all sapped her spirit. She was ready to give up her treatment, even though it was effective.

Her annual celebratory trips with the girls, when she was in remission, had been full of life. Flashing or mooning strangers out of the car window on the way home from these events had been her irreverent way of showing that she was still alive. When her fighting spirit waned, her husband looked for ways to revive it. Family driving vacations with the kids to the mountains or seashore helped. So did a new yellow VW Beetle that the family really didn't fit in, but was cute. The most inspirational effort was when Stan went all out and took his wife on a romantic trip to Rome to throw a coin into the fabled Trevi fountain, promising someday to return. After this, with renewed hope and energy, Jean returned to continue her treatments and is doing well.

EMPOWER YOURSELF

Conquering the panic stage of being diagnosed with cancer is the first step. It is imperative that you start that process now. In later chapters, you will learn more about further developing a trusting relationship with your oncologist. It's imperative that you have an open mind. Telling your physician, for example, that you will never consider chemotherapy treatments pointlessly removes one important component of cancer treatment. You will also learn how to recognize bias in an oncologist's advice and how to work around it. Don't be led to a decision about treatment that you will later regret. Later chapters will help you to grow out of initial depression toward a "one day at a time, enjoy life to its fullest" attitude.

WHAT'S NEXT

The first step after accepting your illness is choosing an oncologist who will *bond with you* and coordinate your treatment. Too many patients underestimate the value of this important relationship.

Chapter 3

Your Most Important Relationship

How Your Oncologist Measures Up

The relationship you have with your oncologist may be the most important one you establish from now on. It could save your life. Trust is the key word here. And trust will lead you to honesty, which is essential if you are to be informed about and understand your full treatment options. This doesn't mean the doctor has to spend a lot of time with you. It simply means you need to have an understanding, a bond. You need an open, honest, nonjudgmental relationship with your oncologist. You can't have that if either side is lying. And, yes, both sides frequently do.

The patient lies. Forgets about the chest pains or the pack of cigarettes she smoked yesterday. "I'm feeling fine, Doctor."

The doctor lies. "There's nothing I can do," translated, "There's nothing else I want to risk trying."

Lies can kill you.

So can myths.

Myth: Doctors know everything. Your common sense doesn't play a role.

Reality: Although you wouldn't want the responsibility of orchestrating your own treatment, your instincts, experiences, and research can play an important role. A wise oncologist will respect your input—and listen.

16

Myth: All caregivers are going to go the extra mile for you.

Reality: Insurers, health care systems, and researchers may have agendas that differ from yours. Some physicians, especially those in large and/or managed-care environments, may provide only the required treatment. They don't want to buck the system.

Myth: Faraway doctors are better than doctors close to home.

Reality: As you'll see in Chapter 5, even though some of the nation's best oncologists work at major centers, your hands-on care at those centers may be with a series of other, less experienced caregivers. Having a series of doctors is likely to result in impersonal care.

Myth: The legal environment in your state doesn't affect your options.

Reality: Some states are notorious for their medical malpractice lawsuit reforms. Often their state legislatures are heavily influenced by powerful trial lawyers. Even though many excellent physicians avoid these environments, patients in the lawsuit-friendly states have less access to specialized care. Regardless of location, how exposed a physician feels he is to liability worries may affect his treatment decisions and level of aggressiveness.

Myth: The doctor has the same view as you regarding quality of life.

Reality: Some doctors are willing to go to great extremes if that is what a patient desires. Others take a more paternalistic view and make decisions for their patients based on what *they think* they would want if they were in that situation. Your oncologist should respect your view of quality of life and not impose his view on you.

Myth: Good doctors are too busy to see you when you're sick.

Reality: Cancer patients especially need access to their oncologists, and your physician should have a plan to get you into the office when you need him. Oncologists are particularly knowledgeable about complications that can arise in cancer patients. Whenever possible, they should not be replaced by physician assistants or emergency room personnel.

LIABILITY AFFECTS TREATMENT OPTIONS

For most cancers, a variety of treatment choices are available and appropriate. Some are conservative; others more aggressive. If the patient wants access to all but a limited scope of treatment, he must assure the oncologist that the relationship is cooperative and not antagonistic.

Most patients aren't aware that fear of liability exposure affects a doctor's treatment decisions. When an oncologist walks into the room to meet with you for the first time, liability exposure may be a predominant concern. If you do nothing to reassure him, he's probably going to stick to only routine, conservative treatments, which often are not enough.

PROACTIVE, NOT REACTIVE

You've heard horror stories about doctors, and you've heard of great doctors who really care. How do you know which kind you're getting? In all honesty, there are lots of good doctors out there.

A good doctor is *proactive*, not *reactive*. This is somebody who takes charge and gets it done now, somebody who isn't afraid to take the initiative when confronting medical and/or any other obstacles to your care. In short, an advocate.

If you want to go the extra mile and have someone who will be there when the going gets tough, you need a practical, hands-on physician who's able to prioritize problems. You need someone who can share his/her recommendation regarding treatment options, but respect and honor your opinion if you don't agree.

The system is so complicated that it's almost impossible to get through it without the help of someone who leads an effective and committed team. Without this, your care will be haphazard.

As with professionals in any other line of work, doctors come in many different types—local or faraway; committed to their patients or committed to their own lifestyles. Probably twenty percent of the oncologists out there are naturally proactive.

FIRST VISIT OR TRYOUT?

Trying to schedule that first visit can be very revealing. If the doctor's office holds tryouts for patients—and a lot of them do—that should be your first clue. A doctor-patient relationship is only established when the doctor gives you medical advice, usually during the first face-to-face meeting. Sending your records does not establish one, and reading them does not expose the doctor to liability concerns.

One of my patients has lived fifteen years with lung cancer. When her first doctor moved, she searched out different oncologists within one hundred miles. Most said, "Send me your records, and we'll get back to you." No doctor-patient relationship was established. The doctors she contacted didn't want a difficult case.

Tryouts can be based on whether you're on Medicare or how pre-treated you are. A cancer patient shouldn't have to try out for treatment. You're picking a partner you'll need to trust with your life. If it's that difficult to be accepted as a patient, this isn't the right doctor for you.

Once you actually meet with the doctor, look for clues in what he is saying that reveal his attitude. A bonded doctor will adopt your problem with language such as: "We need to treat this." "We need to get these films done." The more *we* statements, the better chance of a bond. A doctor who is distant will separate himself by using language, such as: "You need to get this done." "You need to treat this." Does the doctor say *your problem* or *our problem?* Even unconsciously, too many *"you's"* can indicate less involvement in your case.

Body language is also revealing. Does she direct the conversation to you and look you in the eye? Does he speak to your chart or the computer?

Doctor Joe Friday: Just the Facts Ma'am

Helen was an effervescent 66-year-old nursing administrator with breast cancer from a neighboring town. She had spent a lifetime around physicians. After she developed a liver mass, she was sent to a specialized surgeon in a nearby city for evaluation. He was technically excellent, but his personality was abrupt and distant. I recognized and respected his expertise and looked forward to making the best of the encounter. She was coached to be tolerant of his behavioral quirks in order to benefit from his technical expertise.

She arrived at the visit in her usual good mood, prepared for anything. The surgeon in his usual avoidant manner didn't make eye contact and kept his head down as he made detailed notes. "Tell me about your past medical history," he said. Without missing a beat she replied, "I've had four breast biopsies, three colonoscopies, two abdominal surgeries, and a partridge in a pear tree." In an instant, he smiled, made eye contact, and was disarmed.

You can similarly disarm your physician.

WHEN HE'S AWAY

Even the best doctor won't be available all of the time. You need to find out what arrangements he's made for your care when he's unavailable. If you're receiving chemotherapy, you deserve an oncologist who is available to you as often as is possible.

Just because there's a doctor "on call" when your oncologist is unavailable doesn't mean you'll actually get a call back or that he'll deal with the problem if he does call you. All too often, a covering doctor will say something unhelpful, such as, "Well, that's a serious problem. I want you to take it up with your doctor Monday morning."

In your initial meeting, ask what arrangements she's made for being covered. Research the reputation of those physicians. The quality of the team will tell you a great deal about the oncologist and her reputation among her peers.

TRAITS OF A PROACTIVE ONCOLOGIST

Accessibility. How easy is it to get in touch with your doctor? Does he answer calls promptly? If he's planning many long vacations or traveling around the country to give lectures at conferences, chances are he will not be around when you need him. Just because he's working fulltime doesn't mean he's available to his patients fulltime.

Continuity of care matters. There may be times when your condition changes rapidly or there are complications from treatment. At such times, it will be important to be able to get a message to your doctor or be able to see her in a timely manner.

Experience. Ask your oncologist how many cases like yours she has treated in the past. If you know nurses and other medical professionals, ask them how busy the doctor is. A friend in the field can tell you who the most experienced doctors are in your area.

I sincerely believe that it takes five to ten years to learn this job, even with extensive hands-on experience. An oncologist who's seen many cases over many years can quickly make judgments about the complications you're likely to encounter. He knows the best way to explain your condition to family members. He also knows which specialists will give him a definitive answer, and he'll be more confident answering your most difficult questions.

You should be able to find out if your oncologist is still board certified in internal medicine as well as in oncology. To become board certified, your oncologist needs four years of medical school, three years in internal medicine, and two or three years of specialized training in oncology. Many oncologists join a group of oncologists, whose practice does not include internal medicine cases. However, internal medicine experience is a plus in treating many types of cancer. For example, internal medicine experience helps in caring for a cancer patient who has a heart attack that complicates his lung cancer treatment. It also helps when there's a secondary illness, such as lupus, diabetes, or emphysema.

PROBLEM-SOLVING SKILLS

If you present the oncologist with a problem, and she spits back a canned answer, that's not good. For example, a lung cancer patient may complain of shortness of breath. If the doctor retorts, "That's your cancer," without probing further, it's not a good sign. In truth, the shortness of breath could be a blood clot in the patient's lungs, pneumonia, or even a heart attack.

Your doctor should be able to figure things out with you—not just medical problems, but problems of logistics and financing as well. Perhaps you lack transportation to get to the clinic. A proactive doctor will be able to refer you to a group that volunteers to drive people to the hospital. If he's not willing to take the extra time to help you with such relatively simple matters, how do you know he will do so if your condition becomes problematic?

COMMON COURTESY

You'd be surprised how often simple politeness is not observed in doctors' offices. You're both human. Your doctor should greet everyone in the room, acknowledging their presence. He should also:

- Be able to look you in the eye with candor and clarity.
- Ask for and welcome your questions, giving you enough time so that he can provide a complete answer that fully satisfies you.
- Examine you carefully and frequently.
- Be open to a difference of opinion regarding treatment strategy.

- Not be offended if you request a second opinion.
- Allow you to record a consult if you choose.

It's extremely important that you not feel intimidated by this person. The whole process you're experiencing is scary enough, and if you go to someone who blurts out something accusatory like, "What were you doing smoking cigarettes all of those years?," you won't feel comfortable honestly sharing very personal information with him.

REASONABLE WAIT TIME

A small percentage of doctors are habitually late, but the many emergencies oncologists face daily make it difficult for them to stick to rigid schedules. If, however, your waiting times are often more than an hour, you should discuss it with the office staff.

Most of the time, a longer-than-usual wait in your doctor's office can be a sign that she has prioritized the sickest patients first. You wouldn't want a doctor who valued her schedule over a patient's crisis. It *is* an oncologist's office. The very nature of her job demands flexibility. Understanding your doctor's priorities should reassure you about the type of care you will receive.

PATIENT MAKEUP

Is the oncologist's waiting room full of only healthy, well-dressed people? That could mean he takes only the less complicated patients who don't require much of his time. If the waiting room is full of sick people, disabled people, people in wheelchairs, or people carrying medical equipment, then you know you have found a doctor who accepts the mission of taking care of *all* people, including the difficult cases. You may have also found a doctor who will truly care for you, regardless of your economic or medical situation.

ABILITY TO BOND

If a doctor's manner toward you is cold and stiff, it doesn't necessarily mean that he doesn't care about you. More likely, his fear of a possible impending loss limits his ability to get close to you, the patient. Only by bonding and building trust can an oncologist give the most effective care. Over time, even the coldest relationships can warm up when they are nurtured. You want a doctor who recognizes that establishing trust in the relationship is a first step toward your accepting his advice.

Susan and Titus: Two Melanomas, Different Results

Susan, 40, never really gave her physician a chance to develop a trusting relationship with her. She began with a jaded view that doctors were all out for money and that she could achieve the same results with fewer side effects by using herbal supplements. As a result, she turned down a very promising melanoma treatment.

Neither Susan nor her physician realized how developing a bonding relationship over time could help her accept effective therapy. Neither tried. The discussion to initiate treatment never took place. Susan died within three months, completely untreated.

Titus, 58, a wheat farmer and melanoma patient, was also reluctant to receive conventional therapy. Over the course of several weeks, I was able to bond with him and gain his trust. He eventually agreed to what turned out to be a very successful research study. A year later, Titus is still alive and in remission. He is participating in a research study that permits him the latest therapy. When his wife brings homemade bread made from their own wheat to our office, I am reminded of how far he's come in both his care and our relationship.

RESPECTABILITY

It's important that your oncologist gets along with and is respected by other physicians. To develop the best team of caregivers, he needs a network of other top medical specialists with whom he's worked closely in the past. You'll be able to gauge the respect other doctors have for him by how quickly you're scheduled and how well you're treated. By selecting a well-respected oncologist, you automatically inherit a team of outstanding specialists as well.

LEVEL OF COMPASSION

At this point in your life, you are the center of the universe. If your oncologist doesn't have compassion, you need to find another doctor. By compassion, I mean that this person is proactive and committed to giving you the best care without concern for personal gain.

Part of this compassion is being resilient enough to treat you, the new patient, as if you were the only patient that day. You shouldn't suffer because your oncologist has emotional baggage left over from a bad encounter during the day. He may have just lost a patient or been frustrated by an insurance problem, but that should not affect his hope for and interest in you.

What is the level of focus the doctor brings to the visit? Is she concentrating on your questions? Is she interested enough in the relevant details of your case to dig for the truth? Her conversation should be flexible enough to revolve around you. She should be able to address her questions to your level of sophistication and education, as well as to your emotional state. Good oncologists know that patients may need to have information explained to them several different times and ways. It's her job to reassure you, to sense where you are.

Maybe you've known doctors who were distant, even cold. But they were great doctors, right? Not in my opinion. Part of being a great physician is being there for the patient. The doctor shouldn't be a prima donna. He should be a caring professional.

HOW YOU CAN ENHANCE DOCTOR-PATIENT TRUST

As in any relationship, trust is a two-way street. Your doctor is relying on you to demonstrate certain trustworthy behaviors as much as you are relying on him. Here are some ways you can enhance that all-important trust.

PRACTICE ACTIVE LISTENING

Make the communication as strong as it can be by repeating back to the oncologist what you think that he is saying. If you walk out of the room and neither of you has voiced your concerns or your questions, problems will occur. The doctor may be certain that you are going to follow the treatment plan, and you may have decided that you don't think your symptoms warrant doing so. By repeating the doctor's statements and voicing your opinion about them, you are showing respect, which enhances the trust and cuts down on the communication lapses.

AVOID NITPICKING

It's not unusual for a patient to feel irritable. Complaining about waiting time, the temperature of the room, or the time it took to call in routine prescriptions may jeopardize this important relationship. If your doctor is covering the basics in providing good care for you, be gracious enough to forgive minor complaints.

DON'T LET A THIRD PARTY DIRECT YOUR CARE FROM AFAR

Every once in a while, I see a patient in my office who has a family member who is actually making the decisions about direct care—for example, a daughter who lives in another state. That interferes with my ability to connect with you, the patient. There are two of us in the room, and neither one of us is in charge.

If a family member has strong opinions or will be influencing your decisions, have that person call or see your doctor directly. Then he'll know to whom he's speaking and will be able to offer clear communication. Taking this important step will also relieve the local family member who has been put in charge of updating the out-of-town person. Regardless of the level of concern, there's no substitute for your oncologist.

KEEP YOUR DOCTOR IN THE LOOP

It's fine if you feel you need a second opinion or an outside consultation, but keep your doctor informed about what you are doing. One reason is that a second opinion or outside consult may add new information that can be integrated into your care.

Tammi: Secret Second Opinion

Tammi was a 55-year-old woman who had a newly diagnosed ovarian cancer. She hadn't been to the physician's office in over 35 years.

Her family had also not had much experience with physicians or the medical community. When she developed a mass in her groin, she sought the opinion of professionals at her local clinic; they referred her for an evaluation. I was the second of three oncologists she had seen in a week. In addition to the panic she was experiencing, she was unfamiliar with how the medical community worked. We asked her to consider a clinical trial that added an interesting new biological drug to the standard treatments, and she agreed. The treatments were to last a week. On the second day, her sister called in saying that she would be absent for a week with no explanation. While we were left in the dark as to her status, we and the clinical trial system held her position in the study open as long as we were permitted. A week later, with no explanation, she returned and agreed to pick up where she left off.

Two weeks later we received the consultation letter from the major cancer center where she had been seen during the time she was absent. They had agreed with the clinical trial on which she was being treated. Why had she not been comfortable keeping us in the loop? Keeping your doctor informed is essential to your relationship. As you will see, if a patient only wants a second opinion, it is always quicker and more complete if it is arranged through your oncologist.

Another reason is the simple matter of trust. If your oncologist finds out about your consultation after the fact, your relationship will be damaged, possibly irreparably.

Show Up for Your Appointments

This may sound obvious, but you'd be surprised how many patients miss their appointments. If you don't show up at the scheduled time, even the concerned doctors will feel you don't take their time or your care seriously. Conversely, if you arrive prepared for your appointments, with relevant information, forms, or questions, your doctor will be that much more conscientious and prepared in return.

FOLLOW YOUR TREATMENT PLAN

Your oncologist's job is to design and supervise the treatment plan he believes will be in your best interest. Your job is to follow his instructions. Respectfully questioning your doctor's advice enhances trust. Not showing up for a previously agreed on treatment doesn't. If you don't show up for chemotherapy, you are not giving the treatment a chance. Furthermore, you're indirectly telling your doctor that you don't respect his advice. The same is true if you don't complete your CAT scan, physical therapy, or full course of medication.

TAKE NOTES ON YOUR BODY

Specifically reporting your symptoms assists your doctor in diagnosing what's wrong. Such symptoms may include fatigue, unexplained weight loss, pain, blood in your urine, or a lump in your breast.

Too often a patient will tell me his diagnosis rather than his complaint. For example, if you report that you are experiencing shortness of breath, it will help me to examine and find the cancer in your lung. But if you tell me you have pneumonia, it will distract me from diagnosing the true problem with your lung. Perhaps you have a pneumonia caused by a lung cancer that is blocking your airway. Try to communicate your symptoms and complaints to your physician. Let him draw the conclusions and make the diagnosis. There may be a diagnosis other than the one you have considered.

Nobody knows your body better than you do. By honestly assessing changes and symptoms, you will be able to help get the best care. As your oncologist learns that he can trust your observations, he will have a greater level of comfort, which could lead to more treatment options in the future.

THE RELATIONSHIP

The bond you have with your oncologist is similar to the one you have with a religious adviser or a good friend. During a crisis or time of intense emotions, a bond can grow quickly and in a short period of time. It is easier to develop that bond when both you and your oncologist share the goal.

Still, you may need to establish the best bond of all with locally available doctors. Physicians who have the service-to-others mentality seem to be fading fast. All too often, they have been replaced by a new breed of doctors who are well trained but are preoccupied with their own entitlement. Their focus often lies more with their own quality of life than with yours. Developing trust with these physicians will take more effort on your part. The next chapter is devoted to ways in which you can foster this relationship. Your developing the best bond that you can with your local oncologist will pay great dividends at times of crisis, even if you choose to also seek advice from more geographically distant experts.

EMPOWER YOURSELF

Trust between you and your oncologist is crucial. And, you definitely play a role in developing or sabotaging that trust. The bond you work to develop will result in your learning about all treatment options. A proactive oncologist will give better care through his experience, courtesy, problem-solving skills, respect, and compassion.

WHAT'S NEXT

You now know the importance of bonding with your oncologist, but you aren't finished yet. Bonding with and understanding the workings of your oncology team will help you see the bigger picture. Here's your opportunity to learn how the staff is organized and what their roles are.

Chapter 4

Cooperation and Consensus
Bonding with Your Oncology Team

Your medical oncologist's office is where you should feel most welcome and where care for your cancer should start. After you are diagnosed, one office, most likely your oncologist's, should serve as your organizational base of operations. A specialized staff is necessary to help the oncologist organize the treatment. Staff includes physician assistants, nurses, pharmacists, social workers, administrators, clerical workers, and nurse aides, among others.

Organizing cancer care in one office has numerous benefits because it allows a better working relationship among the professionals directing care. These benefits include coordinating and prioritizing your treatment, as well as accurate record keeping. For example, your oncologist can arrange for you to see another doctor faster than you can. He arranges for your admission to the hospital as required for radiation therapy, chemotherapy, late side effects from surgery, or other special needs. Your local community oncology office should also help organize care from outside institutions. By arranging appointments, keeping records of consultations, and reviewing consultant's recommendations, this home office can provide continuity and avoid confusion in care.

Without this continuity, you may suffer complications of disjointed care. Details matter. You may not understand the correct sequence of treatments, you may not know to return for follow-up in a timely manner, or you may not have a good understanding of an outside consultant's report. Your oncology office can provide this information.

YOUR ONCOLOGY STAFF

An oncologist needs a large ancillary staff to help care for you. This includes partners, physician assistants, nurses, pharmacists, nursing assistants, and clerical assistants. It is important to understand the roles of each of these support people. Ask organizational questions first. Who handles medication refills? Who handles disability forms? Whom should you call after hours?

As clinics grow larger, administrators and physicians worry that care has become too impersonal. By becoming familiar with someone in each of these roles, you begin the process of personalizing the process. Personalized care is better care. The staff will take a greater interest in you, remember you, and go out of their way for you. Large cancer hospitals also have patient care coordinators or patient advocates to help navigate these strange complex worlds. These people are there to personalize service and hear grievances in response to criticisms that larger centers may make patients feel like a number.

EDUCATION

Teaching someone about cancer treatment is often the job of nurses and physicians' assistants. For the patient, learning about cancer treatment is like starting a class in physics the night before a big job interview. Emotion and panic limit most people's ability to focus and internalize the information presented. Stay calm. Ask to be taught on a day that is good for you. Don't settle for a large packet of reading material if you don't enjoy reading. Ask for audio or videotapes. Ask someone to explain information verbally if you think that might help. Sometimes, patients prefer learning from the experiences of other patients who have been through similar treatments. This approach might be less intimidating and encourage you to ask different questions than you might otherwise ask. This is also a good way to determine how much you know. It is clear that you understand when you are able to teach someone else.

Staff members can help you more if they are aware of how well you understand your cancer and its treatment. You may have preconceived no-tions that are way off base. Many patients have some ideas based on old wives' tales that have stayed with them. Ask questions about the odd recommendations from Aunt Ethel. Or about the recent magazine article concerning a new discovery or alternative treatment. It is better to ask questions about these matters than to refuse useful treatment based on folklore. Many patients have denied themselves effective care by announcing a refusal to consider treatment based on such misunderstandings and misinformation.

OFFICE ATTITUDE

The outlook of your oncology team often reflects the attitude of the oncologist and the system she feels comfortable working with. Your oncologist has chosen this environment. Most are in large group practices, hospitals, or health care systems. In a smaller office, your oncologist plays a prominent role in running the business. She may have a role in your patient care, as well as in answering financial queries, particularly when you may need financial help. In larger cancer treatment centers, busy committees create treatment guidelines that determine procedures for making these difficult decisions. Such committees may strongly encourage the use of specific treatments for common cancers. Having a close relationship with the individual who makes these decisions may help her to see you as a person, not just a chart number. It is far too easy for an impersonal committee in a large system to dismiss an unfamiliar patient who has fallen on financial hard times. A physician who wears both hats is a rare entity these days, but usually is far more empathetic in such matters.

YOUR ATTITUDE

Physicians are not obligated to see you or take you on as a patient. Indeed, patients are occasionally dismissed from a doctor's practice. Some of the reasons seem reasonable, while others do not. It is possible to refuse to see you anymore if you choose to receive all of your chemotherapy or radiation treatments at another facility. Further, argumentative or litigious patients, as well as patients with a history of financial irresponsibility, can at times be released. It is best to address questions respectfully and directly with the practice management if you have financial troubles or operational criticisms. The exam room visit is not the ideal time and place to criticize.

You might receive positive accolades from staff members when you are friendlier, affable, and don't unduly burden them. It is appropriate to ask for help getting in to see the pulmonologist when you are having a difficult time breathing. Demanding that a busy nurse bring you a glass of water or a newspaper is not acceptable. Patients who are inappropriately demanding or attention seeking are less likely to endear themselves to the staff. Try to do for yourself anything you are able to do.

On the other hand, be aware that you will need the help of the staff on many occasions. Filling out complicated forms, planning weeks of long-named tests in distant departments, and working through information on complicated new medication schedules are all good reasons to ask for help.

Most staff members are well intentioned but human. They have good days as well as bad ones. They have families, soccer games, personal crises, and other problems of their own. They are trying to help your physician treat your cancer as best they can. It rarely helps to vent your frustrations at them. It is often obvious when the attitude of the oncology office is patient centered. You want to feel as if you are being treated as if you are the center of the universe. Unfortunately, in rare cases, the office exists for the benefit of the office staff or physician rather than the patient.

Empowered, proactive office staff members are better able to help than those who are frustrated by layers of directives from distant administrators. They lose focus and hope when their good intentions don't get translated into help for patients. Try to observe if the people in your oncologist's office are burdened by needless bureaucracy. You, the patient, are in a much better position to change their world and system than they are. By using the appropriate channels to offer your suggestions, their work may become easier and more helpful to the patients they want to serve. You might help by speaking to someone on the administration staff of the system that is treating you.

TIMING

Speed matters. Time is of the essence. How fast your oncologist's office responds to you is important. If you call with chest pain today, an evaluation should be done. Now. Your physician's office should see you and rapidly order an EKG, a CT angiogram of the chest (to look for a blood clot), lab tests, and a chest X-ray. If you don't hear from someone in the office today, go to the emergency room. If you have a lung cancer that needs a surgeon's evaluation, this should be completed within two weeks. How fast your oncologist's office arranges tests and consultations is an important indicator of the staff's interest in your care. Speed does matter. The best cancer care starts by your admitting and rapidly reporting any problems. Then, your oncologist needs to take charge and quickly address the issues. Mistakes will always happen. Incorrect decisions are made both by you and by your oncologist. How fast you correct them is crucial. By reporting minor problems, you prevent them from becoming major ones. Calling in with questions about your constipation will prevent a bowel obstruction. Reporting that you become short of breath when you climb stairs will diagnose a pulmonary embolism, or blood clot in the lungs, before a collapse and sudden death.

The tempo of the office staff is guided by the physician's personality and attitude. If the oncologist insists, things will get rolling fast. Start your treatment NOW, not next Tuesday when there is an opening in the chemotherapy schedule. Communication is key. Your oncology office should be available to take calls from other doctor's offices daily. This facilitates your care. When a physician refuses to take a call, or delays returning a call, care is delayed. Time matters.

COMMUNICATION

Your oncologist's office should be able to communicate with you on a timely basis. You want an oncologist and staff members concerned enough to occasionally call you. At times, the day after you finish a complicated treatment, they may contact you. Although this is useful, many issues are best dealt with during an office visit, where you can relay your concerns to the physician directly. Telephone medicine, however, has problems associated with it. Complaints are incompletely explained or not properly recorded. In addition, responses may be delayed. Significant management decisions should not be made over the phone through a third party. They should be made face to face with the oncologist. There is little added expense to another office visit for most patients. The cost is worth the better care that results. At times, the concerns relayed on the phone bear little resemblance to the actual issue. A patient calls in with "I want to stop my chemotherapy treatments." What they actually mean could be anything from "I'm constipated" to "I'm taking a trip" or "I'm depressed and need a break." Take the time to actually talk to your doctor. It's worth the trip to see him. Life-threatening misunderstandings are common when management decisions are left to telephone medicine.

RECORD KEEPING: DETAILS MATTER

It is important that the office staff is conscientious and thorough. Haphazard record keeping is common. Does that report have your name at the top or is it someone else's? It is easier for an oncology office to help you if your cancer treatment began in that office. Rarely are lengthy and duplicative records transferred from other offices or facilities thoroughly reviewed, trusted, or even available. X-rays are frequently repeated despite the enormous expense. If you stay with the same office, information is available to your oncologist in an updated, familiar, and trusted form. Therefore, it makes sense to use trusted consultants who have a daily working relationship with your oncologist. Moving records from one office to another in the middle of a treatment plan becomes bureaucratically complex and time consuming. A series of radiation treatments are rarely interrupted and moved to a new facility. Unfortunately, the new privacy regulations have had the unwanted effect of substantially delaying transfer of your records. Caregivers also worry that a patient who switches physicians may be more likely to be unstable, demanding, and time consuming.

Electronic medical records, known as EMR, are commonplace and will soon be required in medical settings. A computer in the exam room greatly facilitates access to lab reports, X-ray studies, and consultant's reports. It also makes your treatment file more accurate and timely. Records are available to many specialists immediately, as files can be shared. The risk, however, is that the office visit will become awkward and impersonal. Trying to reboot or fix a down computer is frustrating for a physician in the middle of a patient visit. Incorrectly entered information is also a problem. I always double check the name at the top of the document.

Records between two different health-care systems are almost always sent by fax or paper—even if both systems have electronic medical records (EMR). A major flaw in the push for EMR is the problem of transferring records between different hospital systems. One reason is the cost of the computer software that allows records to be transferred between different groups. The second is the lack of a unique number or name that identifies each individual. Social security numbers aren't now used for this purpose.

The physician may be tempted to face a computer while talking to you sitting behind him. The interaction becomes less personal and even more dehumanized. It is challenging to scroll through the computer screens, make eye contact, take notes, and talk to the patient simultaneously. Be aware that glitches with the computer can lead to staff frustrations, unavailable records, and a lack of paper backup. It is also easy for the physician to become distracted by the computer. Electronic medical records are subject to the problems associated with many users all learning *how* at their own speed. Also, at times, various clinics and hospitals have different electronic systems that don't talk to each other, leading to even more physician frustration. Comparing CT scans becomes challenging, lab tests are duplicated, and drug records aren't quickly updated. You may ask to be referred to a specialist who is in the same *system* just for the simplicity of record keeping.

Treatments based on computer protocol models can also lead to errors by caregivers unfamiliar with specific chemotherapy protocols. Hands-on calculations from people familiar with specific drug use, in addition to computer protocol calculation, may allow a backup that permits fewer errors than blipping boxes on a screen. This may be most acute in a teaching facility. If your physician is talking to the computer, ask him to turn around and talk to you. Keep your own paper records of important consultations and issues.

TREATMENTS

Chemotherapy and radiation treatments are sometimes administered in the same clinical area in close proximity to where the oncologist is seeing patients. In this manner, your own oncologist is available to attend to you when a drug reaction or medical crisis ensues. In other situations, however, the treatments are given a substantial distance away from the office. Sometimes, they are given in a completely different building supervised by someone you haven't met.

It is very important to know who is available to help if you have a crisis. A physician or midlevel provider (a nurse practitioner or physicians assistant) should be in the building and able to respond to an emergency. It may not always be your oncologist. By having your own oncologist nearby, you'll have someone who knows your clinical history and is better able to quickly help. It is not uncommon for patients to need to be rapidly moved to the emergency room or hospital. You should know what the plans are if such a necessity arises.

You will probably have to come to the treatment clinic on many occasions when you don't also have an appointment to see your oncologist. Questions frequently come up during these visits. Ask them. The only stupid question is the one you don't ask. Misunderstandings about simple matters, such as bowel preps or medications, may become life threatening quickly. Insist on seeing your oncologist if the nurse or midlevel person can't answer your question. *Insist.* It is not unreasonable to ask to see the oncologist between routine visits when you are having a problem. The oncology office during a routine workday will have current, updated information about you, whereas the emergency room later that night will not.

If you are on a clinical trial, the treatment schedule will be far more rigid. Off-study patients enjoy much more flexibility in resolving the conflicting scheduling needs of everyday life, such as vacations, travel, and family and community events. Many treatments can reasonably be scheduled around them. Travel may present several problems. The most substantial issue is not having access to your own physician and records. Dropping into a strange ER in a distant state may lead to haphazard care. In addition, travel itself may lead to other complications such as blood clots and pneumonia. See Chapter 12 for a discussion of the issues involved in traveling during treatment.

WHAT TO WEAR, WHAT TO EAT

Oncology visits are slow ordeals. Hurry up and wait. Wait to see the doctor, wait to get your X-ray, and wait to get treated. You may be sent for many tests, scans, and EKGs, all of which require time. Bring a book or pastime to divert your attention so as to keep your sanity. Patients who become unduly anxious about the wait and who complain get different care. The anxious, complaining patient gets rushed. Physicians don't linger and talk with them. Thus it's difficult to bond. You want the doctor to talk to you. That won't happen if the doctor wants to just rush you through and get to someone who is friendlier.

Plan to spend most of the day. Bring a snack, a drink, and any other physical necessities. If you need medication, oxygen, or hygiene equipment, bring it. Don't be caught without these needs and demand that the staff perform an ad hoc scavenger hunt on your behalf.

Dress for the occasion. Be accessible. Uncomplicated. Some rooms are especially warm or cold, so dress in layers. In fact, PET scan rooms are so notoriously cold that staff members wear sweaters regardless of the time of year. (A PET scan is an example of a scan that helps to assess the growth rate of a cancer by measuring its metabolic activity). Make it easy for the physician to examine you. You don't want the oncologist to overlook the exam due to inconvenience. This part of the visit is critical to his assessment.

Lucas: Chemotherapy Came Last

Lucas, a recently retired police officer, had a plan to enjoy life. He'd moved from the big city to a small town and had arranged for a weekend with friends and family. Although he had lymphoma, he declined chemotherapy treatment late one week because he didn't want to interrupt his weekend barbecue plans. Instead, he opted to come in the following Tuesday. By Monday, he was in the intensive care unit after suffering a massive stroke, which was possibly a preventable complication of his disease. He never recovered. I don't know if chemotherapy on Thursday would have prevented the stroke, but I've learned over the years that the sooner you treat people, the fewer complications there are.

SUPPORT AND FINANCES

Your oncologist's office knows how to open the doors to find support for you. Social workers, patient care coordinators, and volunteers know how to aid with these matters. Government, industry, and private foundation help for cancer patients abound and are largely underutilized resources (see the resources section at the end of the book). Your oncologist's office should know the best ways to prevent finances from becoming an obstacle to your getting necessary drugs and treatments. Local organizations should be visible and known to the staff. These types of groups will be more hands-on and better able to work with such day-to-day matters as transportation and the cost of medication.

Sometimes patients are too proud to ask for help. They should not be. Tell yourself that you are actually doing a service for those who are offering to volunteer. You give them the opportunity to become involved. They need someone to serve. You're it. Simply allow them to help.

The social worker is your window into the world of what appears to be deliberately overcomplicated government programs. The social worker is your guide when Medicare, Medicaid, VA, and disability rules are implemented differently from time to time and state to state. Those administering these programs sometimes need the social worker to remind them that you are the reason such programs exist, too. Your situation may not neatly fit into the boxes on the forms. Your success with them requires persistence, patience, and a little insider know-how. Many of your fellow patients give up too easily when a cold federal bureaucrat rudely denies their claim. They should appeal it. Don't accept that initial NO.

By the way, medical bills can be a headache. If possible, delegate responsibility for your financial matters and medical bills to a friend or relative. Give them the authority to contact the medical office themselves. It is hard to focus on medical bills when you are not working, out of cash, and sick. But taking care of bills is important. An objective third party helper, such as an older sister, is ideal for this role. Let her fight your denials, make those lengthy frustrating phone calls, and calculate your deductibles.

EMPOWER YOURSELF

Don't forget the importance of the office staff and organization. Your attitude, the office staff's attitude and timing, and communication are all needed to properly coordinate your care. Details and timing matter greatly.

WHAT'S NEXT

Your oncologist's recommendations make more sense when you understand the nature of cancer. The next chapter will introduce you to the basics.

Chapter 5

Understanding Cancer
It's Not Just One Disease

G et the most out of your doctor's explanation of what cancer is. Sometimes, this explanation is too technical and filled with excessive medical jargon. Sometimes, it is too limited. Sometimes, the oncologist assumes a level of medical sophistication far beyond where most patients are. If it's not a good day for you—if you're confused or in pain—you need to let the doctor know that and reschedule an appointment. Discussing your illness with your doctor will be fruitless if you are consumed by anger or denial. I've had patients who just couldn't accept their illness, which wasted valuable time when we could have been discussing it.

"There's no way I could have cancer," one patient told me. "Cancer's caused by preservatives, and we've always eaten healthy food. We didn't even have pancake mix in the house."

Cigarettes and a high-fat diet are two of the biggest causes of cancer. Not pancake mix.

True story. A patient was having coffee with a buddy complaining about how lousy he felt. "Why don't you go see a doctor?" his friend asked.

The patient's response was, "A doctor never gave you any good news, did he?"

It's easy to spot denial in someone else, but much more difficult when you're the one who can't accept the truth.

Another patient came to my office very late in her illness because she was trying to treat her cancer with alternative medicine. She came in only because she was in crisis. If you want to experiment with alternative treatments, inform your oncologist. Don't wait until a crisis to establish contact with this important member of your team.

Don't come alone for your initial meeting. When you see the doctor, be sure you are in the right state of mind to accept the diagnosis. Bring the relevant people—your spouse or an adult child—someone with a clear head, who will be able to write down the information your doctor shares with you. Do not bring well-meaning but delusional people who are convinced that you only need to drink carrot juice for a cure.

One of my patients was so busy trying to take notes for her daughter, who was at work, that she could barely hear what I was saying. The daughter wanted to be with her mother for the surgery, but she did not understand the importance of being with her for the diagnosis. Finally, I said, "Stop taking notes and just listen to me. I'll call your daughter on the phone."

You can't get all the information you need to know from one person on one given day. Just because the doctor said it doesn't mean that you've internalized it. You'll be getting information from different sources, including your surgeon, your radiologist, and your primary source, the oncologist. If it's not a good time for the doctor, maybe a different day is better, maybe a physicians' assistant can help you.

We've discussed initial panic in Chapter 1. It can keep you from hearing what is actually said. The one way to know if you really understand what was said is to repeat it to someone else. Repeat your understanding of your condition to a trusted friend or a companion. If you can communicate what your doctor told you, you will know that you understand it. It's unlikely that you will be treated by just chemo, just surgery, or just radiation; you might be treated by all three. Early on, you should talk to all the people who are going to treat you. The surgeon's focus ought to remain on surgery. Let the radiation oncologist give you advice firsthand about radiation. This will protect you from biased opinions.

DIFFERENT TYPES OF CANCER

Oncologists classify cancer by the primary body site—the part of the body where the cancer first develops (colon, cervix, uterus). Most people think cancer is one disease, but in fact there are many different kinds of cancer, each with a different disease pattern, treatment protocol, and prognosis. Breast cancer is a different disease than testicular cancer. Lung cancer is a different disease than endometrial or uterine cancer.

Cancer is a disease caused by an uncontrolled division of abnormal cells in a part of the body. When enough of these cells divide and pile up, they form a tumor. While all cancer cells are abnormal, each person's cancer cells will be abnormal in a different way. Under the microscope, a brain cancer cell looks entirely different from a prostate cancer cell—and both could look different in another person. Many cancer cells look like immature cells that have not yet begun to specialize into cells of a particular tissue. Others are dividing wildly and out of control.

Many of my new patients misunderstand that cancer can travel, for example, from their breast to their liver or lungs, and it will still remain breast cancer. Breast cancer cells are different from lung cancer cells. However, the breast cancer cells may break away from a tumor mass and invade a patient's lung. In that case, the patient will have breast cancer cells in her lung, rather than a new disease called lung cancer.

Let's say you're a blond guy who lives in Kansas. You're blond, Caucasian, with German ancestry, and you speak English. If you move to Shanghai, you will not, all of a sudden, become Chinese. You will still be a blond-haired, white-skinned guy from Kansas. Likewise, a certain kind of cancer is still the same wherever it is located.

SMART CELLS AND DUMB CELLS

Oncologists like to distinguish between smart (resistant) cancer cells and dumb (sensitive) cancer cells. While physicians tend to use the terms sensitive and resistant, I find that patients understand smart and dumb better to describe the development of resistance in cancer cells. Smart cancer cells are the ones that are able to grow even though you have been undergoing treatment. When you are first diagnosed, it's impossible to distinguish between the smart and the dumb cancer cells. Fortunately, dumb cancer cells, which constitute the majority, are the ones that will be very responsive to chemotherapy or radiation. The smart cancer cells, usually a smaller percentage, are the ones that resist or evade treatment. They can linger in the body, where they will continue to divide, sometimes for many years.

Joe: Three Different Cancers

Joe, a 55-year-old bus driver, was originally being treated for prostate cancer. His PSA, a measure of his total body's burden of his prostate cancer, was markedly elevated at over 500. He had an advanced stage III prostate cancer. Stage III prostate cancer is a prostate cancer that has advanced into the pelvis beyond the limits of the prostate gland. During the treatment and evaluation of his prostate cancer, a new separate stage II colon cancer was discovered. Stage II colon cancer means it hasn't spread beyond the wall of the colon. He had two separate tumors simultaneously. Several years after he was successfully treated for both, his follow-up tests found a mass worrisome for cancer in his lungs. Further tests showed a third new cancer, this time lung disease. He had developed three separate primary cancers. His prostate cancer had not spread to the colon and the colon cancer had not spread to the lungs; they were all different.

Joe's clinical course became even more complicated when continued follow-up tests found him to have a mass in a gland near the kidney called the adrenal gland. Biopsy and pathology tests were done. These tests were able to distinguish among the various types of disease. His lung cancer had spread to his adrenal gland. Since this was removed five years ago, he has been off all treatment and has been free of any cancers.

His course demonstrates how each cancer is different and requires separate treatment strategies.

The longer you have a malignancy, or cancer, the better the chances are that you will develop more of the smart, resistant cells that are more difficult to treat. This is to be expected, as the easiest-to-treat cancer cells die first. Some oncologists will simply continue treatment longer, while others will take a treatment break for six to eight months, and then start another round of therapy. Again and again you will hear me say: *Treatment is always most effective the first time around, and the earlier you treat the disease, the better off you will be.*

Do You Live in a Cancer Cluster?

Having a lot of cancer patients in your neighborhood isn't necessarily a bad thing. It may reflect better treatment or better access to care. First, you need to understand the difference between incidence and prevalence. Incidence refers to how many new patients are diagnosed at the same time. Prevalence refers to how many people have a disease at any one time. Usually, in poorer communities, where there is little access to healthcare. high exposure to toxins, and a high degree of smoking and obesity, the incidence of cancer may be high, but the prevalence low. In other words, in poor communities, many people will get cancer and few of them will survive for long.

In more affluent communities, where the population receives and has better access to regular health care, smokes less, exercises more, watches its diet, and lives farther away from toxic sites, the incidence of cancer may be low, but the prevalence high. In other words, in rich communities, fewer people will get cancer but more of them will survive. So it's important to ask whether there are many people who have been living for a long time with cancer—in which case it may *seem* that there is a lot of cancer in your neighborhood—or whether many people in your neighborhood have died from it.

Staging

One of the most important aspects of your diagnosis will be its stage. The stage is how far along your cancer has spread. Each different type of cancer has its own detailed staging system. Your oncologist should explain how your cancer has been staged and what that means for treatment and prognosis. Every cancer tumor begins as Stage 1 and, if left untreated, will move to Stage 2 and then Stage 3. Some cancers move slower or faster than others, but all solid cancers are diagnosed as Stage 1, Stage 2 or Stage 3, or Stage 4. For example, breast cancer remains breast cancer through all three stages. Even if it spreads to your liver, it does not morph into liver cancer. However, it would be called stage IV breast cancer because it has spread so far. Similarly, if lung cancer travels to your brain, it does not become brain cancer. Instead, it is called stage IV lung cancer in your brain. Below are descriptions for each stage.

Stage 1

This is the stage at which cancer is easiest to treat. If you have been diagnosed with Stage 1 cancer, it is not a good idea to wait until it advances to another stage before beginning treatment because you will have missed the opportunity for the most highly effective treatment of the disease.

Denying symptoms that may indicate a Stage 1 cancer or delaying a visit to your doctor can mean you are putting your life at risk. Stage 1 cancer means that the diseased cells are organ confined. Stage 1 prostate cancer means the cancer is confined to the prostate gland. (Stage 1 kidney cancer means the cancer is confined to the kidney.) Although it is favorable to be diagnosed at stage 1, some cancers, such as pancreatic cancer, are rarely detected at this early stage.

Stage 2 and Stage 3

These are stages at which cancer is often still very treatable. A Stage 2 or 3 cancer has begun to spread or is spreading to areas around the initial tumor site. (Stage 2 or 3 prostate cancer means the cancer has spread outside the prostate gland, perhaps to the urethra or bowels. Stage 2 or 3 breast cancer means the cancer has spread outside the breast to the lymph nodes.) The oncologist's concern about stage 2 and stage 3 is whether the cancer has spread to yet other unknown areas and might actually be a stage IV cancer.

Stage 4

This is the stage at which cancer has spread to distant organs. The cancer has metastasized to other parts of the body. While it's not good news to be diagnosed with a Stage 4 cancer, your oncologist can most likely offer you treatment to slow the disease and medicine to ease any pain you may have. Only a small number of stage 4 patients are long-term survivors. One of my patients had stage 4 breast cancer that had spread to her lungs. However, it was in only one area of the lung, and we were able to treat it. Five years later, it has never returned. She was one of the lucky ones.

HOW YOUR STAGE IS DETERMINED

Bear in mind that determining your cancer stage is an inexact science and is usually a best guess or approximation. Cancers that occur inside the body, such as ovarian, colon, or uterine, are often not discovered until they have reached a later stage. Cancers that are more noticeable on your body, such as breast cancer or skin cancer, are easier to discover at an earlier stage.

There are two ways your cancer stage can be described: clinical and pathological.

Clinical Staging is determined nonoperatively through a physical examination, CAT scan, MRI, biopsy, or blood test. The danger with clinical staging is that an oncologist sometimes underestimates how far the cancer has advanced. This is a best guess without surgery. For example, if we see two spots, or lesions, in the liver on a CT scan, it doesn't mean that there are two areas of cancer in the liver. We only know that we can see two. These lesions may be the tip of the iceberg; there may be more areas of cancer that the scans are not picking up. Or, the lesions may appear as cancer on the scans and actually represent benign noncancerous processes. This is because clinical staging is reached only with information that can be *seen*. Therefore, if clinical staging results in the assumption that your cancer is an earlier stage III when it is actually an advanced stage IV, you may be undertreated. It is not uncommon for the assumptions made here to cause major problems.

Pathological Staging is determined after surgery when your surgeon, oncologist, and pathologist, a doctor trained to recognize cancer stages by their appearance under a microscope, can see *inside* your body.

Usually your cancer stage will be determined by a combination of clinical and pathological signs.

One common myth is that being exposed to air will make cancer cells grow. This false belief points to the discrepancy between a clinical and pathological stage. If a surgeon cuts open a patient, thereby exposing his intestines to the air and finds the patient has cancer throughout his abdomen, the cancer has only "grown" because the surgeon operated and found it. The growth is not due to the air in the room!

AM I GOING TO DIE?

This is the first question every cancer patient has, and I can't answer that. No one has a guarantee that he or she will wake up tomorrow. Two thirds of breast cancers that are caught early are cured, and there are cures for many other cancers, as well. Similar to other chronic diseases, such as diabetes, some cancers can be treated but not cured.

Improvements in earlier stage detection and new and/or improved treatments are increasing the survival rate for all cancer patients. Approximately half of all cancer patients now survive at least five years after treatment. People who remain free of cancer during that time have a good chance of remaining permanently free of the disease.

Your prognosis depends largely on how far your cancer has advanced — its stage — the type of cancer you have, and how it will respond to treatment. Kidney cancer, or mesothelioma when it is advanced, may be treatable but will have a low chance of being cured. Other cancers are much more easily cured.

Many people admire Lance Armstrong's cancer survival story. He had a very advanced stage of cancer — advanced to the point where it had apparently widely spread to his lungs and brain. He was treated successfully because the cancer was not brain or lung cancer, but testicular. Lucky for Lance, testicular cancer is very responsive to treatment. Normally, after four weeks of appropriate care, a person has a 90 percent chance at a cure. Armstrong's "miracle" was in fact predictable from the point of view of oncology.

Your doctor should be able to give you a relatively secure prognosis. But he or she cannot look into a crystal ball and tell you how much time you have left. Ask your doctor to give you the statistical survival rates for someone with your type and stage cancer, and then ask him to apply those percentages to your individual case.

BE PROACTIVE

- Use your diagnosis of cancer as an early detection method for other cancers. Also take advantage of close follow-up. Whatever causes a first cancer may cause a second and third cancer. Early testing and close follow-up are crucial to your health.
- Don't put off your diagnosis. Many people come in late, including spouses of patients. For example, if we are treating the husband, he may get all of the attention. Finally, the wife will show up with an advanced cancer because she deferred diagnosis.
- If you don't understand, ask. The oncologist sometimes may speak in jargon. Remember the average medical student learns thousands of new words in school. Interrupt and ask the oncologist to translate so that it makes sense to you.

- Take your time. Your subconscious needs time to digest the information you're receiving. Sometimes it helps to break up the office conversation with patients by discussing family, common interests, or church. Take all of the time you need to assimilate the information.

To understand cancer and the rapidly changing treatments, you need a rapport with your oncologist. No book will be able to keep up with all that we're learning about this disease.

EMPOWER YOURSELF

As you now know, cancer is many different diseases. Your cancer is different from that of your friends and relatives. This explains why your oncologist is confident that it may be far more treatable. By understanding your cancer, its nature and stage, you remove some of the fear and gain knowledge and confidence.

WHAT'S NEXT

You've gotten the diagnosis, and your first thought is to head for one of the major cancer centers, right? The next chapter will show you how to decide if that's in your best interests.

Chapter 6

Major Cancer Centers
What Every Patient Should Know

Many enormous advances in the world of cancer treatment have been spearheaded by comprehensive cancer centers. Many new biologic and chemotherapy drugs, combined modality treatments, and other advances have been moved forward into everyday treatment through the efforts of these major cancer centers. Their physician researchers often have the most up-to-date knowledge of each type of cancer they study. The successful early phase trials at these centers are then studied more thoroughly in larger populations. These are called *cooperative group studies*, and patients who are able to participate in them benefit from the advances firsthand.

Most people assume that if they decide to have second opinions, surgery, chemotherapy, radiation, or other treatments at one of these centers, they need only make certain that their insurance will cover it, call for an appointment, and go. This is not always the case. Major cancer centers sometimes have specific selection criteria and, if you don't meet these criteria, you won't be accepted as a patient or selected for a study. In other words, they pick you, not the other way around.

THE BIG CENTER EXPERIENCE

Overwhelming is the way most patients describe their cancer center experience. This is one time you need a friend. If at all possible, bring your own support person, whether a spouse, family member, or trusted friend. This person can help you remember medical and personal details, run errands and interference, and keep in contact with your family, friends, and colleagues.

Many patients are self-referred, in which case you may need to do more of the legwork yourself. Most important, several crucial hurdles are common to most "big center" experiences. First, the big cancer center physician will not assume that the results from your local doctor or hospital are correct. The big center physician will often order everything redone. He may want to redo or at least reread your CT scans, bone scans, and other tests and labs. He will want to look directly at your biopsy slides. If possible, bring them with you. Don't mail or send them ahead as they may get lost.

Most of the time, your point of contact at the center will be someone other than a physician. Likely you will be offered a meeting with a social worker and often allowed the use of a patient advocate. Be sure to get this person's phone number when you meet with him or her, so you can keep in touch whenever you have questions or concerns. While the center may seem large and impersonal at times, if you search you will always find people who care. The fact that you're offered the resource of a patient advocate suggests, however, that others have faced challenges within this system.

The efficiency of the clinic varies tremendously. Each department or office has its own methods and style. Clinics that treat rare tumors, such as sarcoma or brain tumors, seem more organized than clinics overwhelmed by many patients with common cancers, such as breast or colon cancers.

The big cancer center experience usually involves a great deal of waiting. A two- to four-week wait for an appointment is common. During this time, your insurance and financial status will be checked to determine your eligibility. A preliminary review of your case by phone or record review may also take place to ensure that you are in the right clinic. For example, does a patient with a sarcoma in her breast get seen in the breast cancer section or in the sarcoma section?

After you arrive, expect to wait at least a week to get all of your scans, physician visits, and lab tests done. Some complicated cases will take more time. Certain cancers are more amenable to this waiting time. Others are not. Significant tumor progression can occur during this waiting period for advanced small cell lung cancer and pancreatic cancers, for example.

STUDIES AND CLINICAL TRIALS

Physicians working at cancer centers are strongly encouraged to treat patients under the auspices of a clinical trial. Their career advancement partially depends on their ability to put people in clinical tests and then publish the results. Much advancement in cancer treatment has been made through them. However, your survival will depend on how rapidly and accurately you can sort through your best options.

A common misconception is that if you have tried everything else, a clinical trial is the answer. In reality, many studies are done primarily on treatment-naïve patients, that is, patients who have *not* been previously administered to. If you apply to a center and are not selected for the study because you are too weak or have other medical problems, you may lose valuable time being evaluated rather than starting necessary treatment elsewhere.

SELECTION BIAS

Patients who have been heavily pretreated or who have previously been through a major cancer surgery often have difficulty getting accepted for such trials. One frequent criticism of studies originating in large cancer centers is that results may be more positive because of selection bias. Previously untreated cancer patients respond best to cancer treatments. This is part of the reason why the number of patients who respond to successful treatment regimens may diminish once these studies are moved from the larger single center trials into larger, community-based clinical trials.

Features of your condition that may allow you to be considered for a study are called inclusion and exclusion criteria. Inclusion criteria include having a particular type of cancer at a certain stage or requiring that the areas to which the cancer has spread, or metastasized, be measurable. Exclusion criteria limit study participation to patients with good kidney, lung, liver, and other important organ function, which are strictly measured by lab tests and X-rays. Pregnancy is a common exclusion.

Exclusion criteria might restrict people whose liver blood levels are high because of a history of hepatitis or alcohol abuse. Exclusion criteria might also limit anyone who has lost more than ten percent of his/her body weight, a problem frequently found in advanced lung, pancreas, and colon cancer patients. Lung cancer patients usually have other tobacco-related problems, such as heart disease, hypertension, or kidney problems, that may exclude them.

To carefully address a specific scientific question, a researcher can limit a study to only uncomplicated cases. This is done by careful selection of the inclusion/exclusion criteria. While it's understandable why a researcher would do that for the benefit of a research study, in the short term, it doesn't help many of the patients in search of treatment. Because studies often focus on those patients with the best health and organ function, there is less information available on how to treat patients with more complicated illnesses, poor organ function, or multiple cancers.

LOGISTICAL CONSIDERATIONS

Major cancer centers may be obligated only to see those patients in a certain geographic area. Patients outside it are selectively accepted based on a variety of factors. To get around this, some patients have even undertaken the expense of renting an apartment in or near a center just to ensure admission.

Rushing off to one of these centers on receiving a cancer diagnosis might not be the best decision for you, however. I have seen many patients succumb to their tumors or other complications while waiting to be seen at such hospitals.

Likewise, relocating to a cancer center increases stress and disruption to your life and your family. Enormous personal and financial resources are required to keep the long-distance cancer treatment going, even when similar therapies may be available to you locally. Often, by the time you return home, financial resources, medical leave, and the patience and support of your family are exhausted. *Caregiver Fatigue Syndrome* develops rapidly. When this exhaustion is combined with the despondency of leaving a major cancer center without successful or anticipated results, a patient may, in turn, decline further therapies. Even though other treatments may be helpful, the combined exhaustion prevents their being used.

Leta: The Price of Postponed Treatment

Leta was a 65-year-old woman with a mass in her pancreas. She began dropping weight, and her health was deteriorating. Her son and daughter-in-law panicked. Leta's general family doctor, still in search of a diagnosis, continued to order tests, but the situation was getting beyond their grasp. With the best of intentions for their mother's care, the family requested that Leta be sent immediately to a comprehensive cancer center. The family's fear over Leta's rapid decline in health precipitated a knee-jerk decision in favor of a cancer center because they believed, as most people do, that their mother would be in the best and most immediate hands possible. The family doctor complied with that request.

Once at the cancer center, Leta went through a month's worth of evaluations. Although the hospital quickly made the diagnosis of pancreatic cancer, the treatment options were not straightforward because of the onset of jaundice caused by her disease.

Believing that a clinical trial was in her best interest, the center attempted to help Leta become eligible for the study. This included many protracted efforts to reverse her jaundice, which proved unsuccessful. As a result, this jaundiced condition rendered Leta ineligible for the clinical trial. She was dismissed from the hospital with no plan, no communication, and no hope. During the long evaluation period, her condition deteriorated, and caregiver resources were depleted. Any option for a reasonable alternate treatment plan was no longer viable. Leta's window of opportunity had closed three weeks before I saw her. Although her family acted out of the best of intentions, their decision resulted in the loss of precious time that could have, instead, been used effectively toward Leta's treatment. Sadly, she passed away shortly thereafter.

Before applying for a clinical trial, it's important to understand one cold, hard reality: the purpose of that trial is primarily to evaluate the success of a new drug/treatment, which may not necessarily cure you. Most patients perceive that they're going to get a better drug or a better therapy because what's being tested is cutting edge. Unfortunately, some patients in clinical trials find that their condition deteriorates rather than improves.

The first things to ask yourself and then discuss with your oncologist are: Why do you want to do this? Is it because you and your oncologist truly think it is best for you or because a friend or family member is insisting? Will the study improve your chances of recovery? You should carefully discuss these and other questions you might have with your oncologist. Can you afford the expense? Although you won't be charged for the drugs, you will be billed for everything else and, if your insurance considers the cancer center "out-of-network," it will cover less, leaving you to pay for most of the treatment, as well as all of your travel costs.

CLINICAL TRIALS: UNDERSTANDING THE PHASES

Clinical trials are carefully designed patient studies helping to advance treatment by addressing research questions. Many studies are available. Some are sponsored by federally funded cooperative groups, while others are sponsored by pharmaceutical companies. Once a study is designed and begun, it is difficult and unusual to alter the treatment plan substantially even if other, and possibly, more effective treatment is subsequently developed elsewhere.

In conditions that are easy to handle, such as strep throat or a headache, physicians administer drugs with no noticeable side effects. However, because cancer is difficult to treat, patients in trials are given doses of drugs at the highest levels possible. As a result, researchers must carefully study patients' responses to those drugs to determine the highest dose that a human being can tolerate without fatalities.

Clinical trials occur in three phases: Phase I trials are generally offered only at larger cancer institutions, while Phase II and III studies may be available in other settings. Contrary to what most people believe, clinical trials don't progress from Phase I to II to III. A study is listed as a certain phase based on the type of scientific question being asked and which drugs are being used.

Previously untreated cancer patients are best suited for Phase II or III studies. Those who have had many previous treatments are often directed toward Phase I studies. Certain groups require special considerations. Prisoners, for example, are ineligible for clinical trials. Patients with psychiatric diagnoses may be eligible for studies as long as they are capable of giving informed consent to the study. Clinical trials study all aspects of cancer care. This includes integrating various treatments in varying degrees, such as surgery, radiation, and chemotherapy drugs. Most studies build on the current standard of care. Patients in randomized studies will receive at least the current standard of care, often better.

Phase I. You can enroll in a Phase I study even if you have previously participated in other studies. They are open to any cancer patient who has not responded to standard treatment. As this treatment is often a last resort, the vast majority of patients participating in Phase I studies ultimately succumb to their disease.

Because the drug administered in a Phase I study has never been tested in humans and the proper dosage has yet to be determined, the primary goal of this stage is to evaluate the toxicity and side effects of the drug. The first patients treated may receive doses so low that the benefits are inconsequential. Later patients will receive increased dosages until the drug causes undue toxicity. A few patients, unfortunately, are treated with doses that are so high that they cause excessive side effects. These reactions may be reversible or they may be permanent and, possibly, fatal. Once an effective dose is determined, it becomes the starting point for a Phase II study.

Phase II. Once researchers determine the highest tolerable dose of a new drug for the majority of patients, the next step is to measure its effectiveness. All patients in a particular Phase II study receive the same treatment. It could be a type of chemotherapy, biological therapy, or course of radiation. Patients in the study must all share the same type and stage of the disease and be previously untreated.

If you're considering taking part in a Phase II study, try to research how other patients have fared on the drug. If you find that other patients with your type of cancer were treated with it, the toxicity is manageable. If the patients are doing well, this may be an advantageous study for you. In certain rare situations, a Phase II study drug can be more effective for you than the standard treatment available for your type of cancer.

Phase III. To get a drug approved, it must be proven superior to other available therapies. Phase III trials are designed to compare a new and hopefully superior treatment to what is standard. It doesn't necessarily have to offer a cure, but the people who take it must show improvement by some measure. In other words, the drug should foster longer survival, a longer remission, and better quality of life than existing approved drugs.

Phase III studies are the gold standard used to clarify the success of the treatment. They may encompass other treatment forms besides drug therapy. For example, several Phase III studies helped to clarify the limited usefulness of bone marrow transplants in breast cancer patients. For many years, autologous bone marrow transplants were studied at many comprehensive cancer centers. The transplants were thought to be superior to conventional chemotherapy in helping high-risk breast cancer patients avoid recurrences. When these Phase III studies were undertaken, the findings showed that these transplants did not necessarily result in greater improvement over the conventional treatments of routine chemotherapy. As a result, resources that had been expended in transplant studies were diverted to more effective therapies. Large cooperative group systems and the Veterans Administration hospitals are able to administer and run these phase III studies.

David: Miracles Do Happen

Miracles happen, and patients do get lucky. David was one of those. A 72-year-old prostate cancer patient, he'd had cancer for ten years and had gone through surgery, radiation, and hormone therapy. When Dave went to a large cancer center, it was to take part in a Phase I study, which as you've seen above, is a study in which a drug is being used in humans for the first time.

As previously noted, Phase I studies are risky, but David had few options left to try. In his case, the response has been very dramatic. His symptoms are no worse, he's not on as many pain medicines, and he is able to travel. For him, it paid off.

Things to Do (Other Than Panic)
During a Cancer Center Evaluation

Your experience at a big cancer center will likely involve days, not just hours, of waiting around in a strange place and city. Although the main reason you are there is for your medical evaluation and subsequent treatment, keeping your mind busy with useful activities can help you avoid despondency while waiting for the decision. Here are some activities to help you pass the time:

- **Take advantage of lectures and educational opportunities.** Big centers often have daily lectures on many subjects of concern to patients. Get the e-mail addresses of the speakers and keep in contact with them. They may have important networking contact information you can use in future.

- **Research your disability and other benefits** available through your employer.
- **Discover the extent of financial help available to you** through foundations, state organizations, pharmaceutical companies, military programs, Veterans Administration programs, and other institutions. Large cancer centers often have a complete listing of the types and amount of help for which you are eligible.
- **Get a listing of the most relevant Web sites** for your particular type of tumor. The staff at the center may know of important Web sites, blogs, and e-mails for key contacts.
- **Research an alternative treatment center.** You could sort through the center's data to see if there is an opportunity for increased hope. Have any formal studies been completed?
- **Ask to see a physical or occupational therapist** about your condition *before* you get a complication. For example, education from a lymphedema physical therapist for breast cancer patients can educate you as to the best exercises to prevent arm swelling.
- **Get a third opinion.** Consider getting another physician's opinion from another nearby cancer center. This could be a more honest opinion about your situation and not just the official party line.
- **Contact your member of congress** to assist you if you are having problems with Federal programs, such as Medicare, Medicaid, or the Veterans Administration.
- **List your available financial resources** to help you in your effort against cancer.
- **Make a tally of personal resources,** friends, religious and community organizations that you can call on. Keep a list of contact information in the event that you need help, such as a ride home from the airport when you are worn out.
- **See a dietician.** Learn what foods may help to limit edema, constipations, bowel blockages, blood sugar changes, and other complications.

- **Keep compiling your own health record,** including copies of important CT or MRI scans for future physicians.
- **See a psychologist.** As your life changes, body image changes and issues of sexuality, work, and self-esteem come up. While you may eventually want to resume this discussion with a more permanent connection back home, get the process started at the center, even if it's just one visit. Psychologists at large centers have seen many patients in similar situations and are able to help you adjust.
- **Fight depression** by learning a new method of relaxation. Meditate. Pray. *Eat.* As hard as it may be, use the time available to enhance your energy.
- **Discover new and exciting flavors.** Cancer patients often experience altered taste sensations. This may be the time in your life when unfamiliar cuisines taste good.
- **Talk to another patient** in the waiting room. Developing even a brief friendship can bring comfort. Families become close. Exchanging visits can become a mutual wellness goal.
- **Keep a journal.** This may allow you to explore your thoughts in this time of great change in your life. Making a journal is sometimes cathartic. It may also be helpful to family and children to know what your thoughts were as you went through challenging times.
- **Delegate important tasks to friends** who have asked if they can be of help. Your sister in another state may not be physically close, but she is able to sort through bills and insurance statements. Having someone take over this and other taxing chores can be liberating. Use your precious time for more relaxing activities. You may have heard this before, but it is important to allow others to help.

In short, don't just wait during the two or four weeks you may be at the center. *Live.* Think of positive things you can do with the precious time available.

GET A DIRECT OPINION

Tumor boards are frequently used in big cancer centers to review plans for patients who require several different types of treatment. They're meetings of physicians of different specialties and are usually held at universities. These weekly discussions groups may include surgeons, medical oncologists, and radiation oncologists, as well as such other specialists as urologists or head and neck surgeons. The tumor board may focus on one particular type of cancer, such as lung cancer. A physician from one department, such as a surgeon, may give the group information about your condition. The other physicians present review this information and offer their opinions about what treatment plan is best. Often, a note is made summarizing the discussion.

However, it is best that the opinion you receive come from a physician who has interviewed and examined you directly. At times, patients are examined by one physician, for example, a surgeon or a medical oncologist, and then the other doctors offer treatment opinions based solely on indirect information reviewed during a tumor board conference. This may not be optimal, as one doctor may glean information from an interview and examination that another did not. One physician may have assumed that your back pain was from the old injury, while another may have wanted to do further testing to determine if the cancer had spread there. One doctor may use leading questions, whereas another would have used more open or honest questions. You are OK with the surgery aren't you? Is a different question than, "What are your thoughts about the option of surgery?"

Physicians may also feel less intimidated about giving an honest opinion when they are discussing your case with you alone face to face. You deserve to hear the specialist's opinions directly. Don't agree to a plan unless you've spoken with all of the specialists essential to your case. Insist on a face-to-face consultation with physicians representing all the specialties important to your case. Don't settle for a phone call or a discussion with an assistant. This information is too important. Ask them the difficult questions. Be firm, but polite. This may take some time, but it's worth it. It should be expected that patients traveling some distance to be seen at a major cancer center will need to be seen by two or three different types of specialists

At times, doctors may use telephone consultations to make their sad duty easier. It is often very challenging to tell someone unfortunate news.

The impersonal phone call could be a technique to avoid this. I have found it reassuring to always discuss important news face to face. This limits misunderstandings that can confuse patients and make bad news even worse. Talking face to face also allows the oncologist time to read the patients nonverbal body language.

CONTINUING CARE AT HOME

Many times, unless you specifically ask to have your follow-up treatment at home, it will be assumed that you want your care to be at the big cancer center. A patient receiving radiation therapy for a throat cancer may legitimately be asked to receive the treatment at a center far from home by a radiation oncologist who specializes in throat cancer. But receiving the radiation therapy for one or two months at a center five hundred miles or more away from home may be too taxing on your family and resources. You should be treated where it makes the most sense for you to receive your care. Marketing should not play a role in where you receive your care.

Patients sometimes pay exorbitant out-of-network bills at a distant large center unaware that identical treatment exists at home. If you ask, your follow-up care can possibly be coordinated between the hometown and big center physicians to allow the same treatment locally. It is rare that a treatment is possible at only a large hospital. If you have a rarely utilized or complicated treatment regiment you may need to ask which local oncologists are most comfortable helping give your treatments.

Whether you're in a big center, HMO, or a private physician's practice, you should know that a large percentage of the revenue in medical oncology comes from intravenous drug profits. Groups that buy a larger number of medications make a larger profit than groups that buy a smaller number. This is because larger groups get a much bigger discount on the purchase price of such drugs. Thus, while all oncologists in a region may be paid at the same rate by Medicare for a specific treatment, their profit is determined by how much the drug costs them to acquire.

A large cancer center operates within tight budget parameters, so their system is at its most financially efficient with a larger volume of patients. Extra costs are expended because of research and teaching. Because of this, the doctors at centers are not always highly motivated to find solutions that allow a patient's treatment to be coordinated closer to home.

Ask questions. You've got to advocate for yourself. Many resources exist at these centers, but it is usually the self-advocating patient who gains access to them. Inquire about help with finances, time off from your job, travel expenses, and coordination. When you ask for help, do so in the same cooperative—not antagonistic—manner that you would use when communicating with your own oncologist's staff. Most people respond better to courtesy than to demands. But be firm.

THE IMPORTANCE OF YOUR LOCAL ONCOLOGIST

I firmly believe that most of your care should be provided as close to home as possible. Home is where you are at your most comfortable, and where the emotional and spiritual support of your family, friends, and community is at its strongest and most accessible. Having a hometown oncologist you trust will give you important advantages, even if you opt for treatment at a cancer center.

As your local oncologist is most likely someone recommended by your family physician, you have the comfort of knowing that you will have access to your medical history as well as the ability to confer with someone who knows you well. This can provide peace of mind during a challenging time. Regardless of the path of care you pursue, particularly if you pursue treatment at a major cancer center, your local oncologist can advise and assist you with options and explain matters in ways you can readily understand. He can provide important and necessary information regarding that treatment and help you apply for a clinical trial. Most important, he can act as liaison with the cancer center before, during, and after your course of therapy. Once you return home from a center, your local oncologist will also monitor you to ensure that your health remains stable. If any concerns are raised, he'll be of prompt assistance.

Your local oncologist can also perform an initial screen to see if you have adequate liver, heart, and kidney functions to be on a study. He'll know the status of your tumor and how the timing of treatment can positively (or negatively) impact your results. He may also be aware of an appropriate clinical trial being conducted close to home and will know if you appear to meet most of the entry criteria. Keeping your oncologist in the loop will reassure you that someone knowledgeable about your treatment is available locally in case of emergency.

Your oncologist can also assess the risk of delaying your treatment during lengthy staff evaluations and serve as an independent advocate within the system. He can be your best ally in case you don't make the cut at the big center. If you do, he can provide pertinent medical information to the center's physicians to ensure the best possible treatment.

It often takes weeks or months to come to terms with a cancer diagnosis and all its ramifications for you and your family. Your grieving process goes through several stages (denial, anger, bargaining, and depression) on your way to eventual acceptance of your disease. Your local oncologist is more committed to your welfare. He knows how the emotional process works. He will likely help you and your family face the reality of your illness and its prognosis. He'll also be able to aid in a way that a doctor at a center—who has no personal history with you and meets you at your weakest and most vulnerable - cannot.

Many patients don't even want the oncologist to know that they're going to a big center. This is a mistake. Ask yourself why you don't want to involve your local oncologist. Are you seeking a treatment that your doctor will consider unreasonable? Do you feel that your doctor is unavailable to you?

It's important to select a proactive oncologist. If yours is not, find another who is. Explain why you want to go to the big center and ask your doctor to help you determine the pros and cons of this decision. However, because of the complexity and rarity of certain malignancies, your oncologist will likely agree that multidisciplinary treatment is best done in concert with a major cancer center. She can work with you to get you the best treatment possible.

PHYSICIAN ACCESS AT THE CANCER CENTER

You may be selecting a large hospital because you believe you're going to be seen by an expert in your particular type of cancer. If you make it through the selection process, that could happen. If you are not selected, you will probably be informed of the news by someone junior on the medical team, someone with less experience than your hometown oncologist. Most disconcerting to you, the message could be short, abrupt, and unduly pessimistic.

Your doctor at the large center may not be available all of the time because in addition to handling specialized cases, he also attends meetings and out-of-town conferences. Senior physicians may not be expected to take calls or to answer day-to-day questions about complications and developments. This results in many issues being addressed by staff physicians, nurses or physician assistants.

Joe: Missing Expert Physician

Joe was a 67-year-old retired executive with leukemia. His disease had been developing over the last several years with intermittent ups and downs in his chronic course. At the urging of his family and for his own peace of mind, he sought out a second opinion at a major cancer center. When time came for the appointment, he enjoyed visiting with the expert and planned a follow-up visit six months later. At these follow-up visits, he would intermittently be seen by the expert physician and occasionally by a physician's assistant if the doctor was unavailable.

One week when Joe was back at home in the waiting room anticipating a visit with me, he was rather surprised to see the large cancer center expert walking through. Joe had just returned a day or two before from a visit to the large center where the physician's assistant had performed the visit alone. The physician was unavailable, he was told. The expert had arrived in our state to give a lecture, which was sponsored by a large pharmaceutical company.

It is understandable that many specialists help by giving lectures to others and that the assistance given by the pharmaceutical companies is appreciated. Their physician assistants are also well experienced and trained. It would seem appropriate however, to insist that you always be seen by the doctor's and not by the assistant only.

When you realize that the aims of the large cancer centers may differ from your goals and those of your local oncologist, it makes sense to reconsider your options and explore all avenues of treatment before making a commitment. Most important, always keep your local medical resources at hand.

Judith: Clinical Study but
No Hometown Connection

Judith came through the emergency room one night when I was on call. Her symptoms included fever, chills, low blood count, and passing out. She'd had a lymphoma for six or seven years. Although she was of modest means, she had enrolled in a clinical study that included travel funds for her to a major clinic. You can find out about such trials in many ways, for example, through your community oncologist, various disease-related Web sites, or directly from physicians involved in this medical research. Travel/living expenses are often major hurdles for patients, so Judith considered herself fortunate.

Her pattern was to travel to the clinic, get treatment, and return to work without seeing a local doctor. Her only contact was a research nurse at the large clinic. As she got weaker, she was told to take higher and higher doses of medicine. Judith had been phoning four states away, unaware that she was calling a research physician's office without 24/7 coverage. Not having a specialist always available was a violation of a study. She was sick, and they hadn't responded. We notified the study coordinators so that Judith would be properly attended to when she returned.

Most people don't have that coordination between the home oncologist and the cancer center. The big center may not have "after hours." It's unwise to have your only relationship be with someone there. You need another connection, preferably one close to home.

RETHINK THAT LAST RESORT

When the body is weakened and time is running out, the large cancer center can offer hope that the patient and family so desperately need. Turning to the large center as a last resort, however, can be as problematic as making it your first stop. As stated earlier, you can and probably will lose precious treatment time as you're being tested and evaluated.

In my experience, most families regret taking their loved ones to a large center as a last resort. A common motive is to allay the survivor's guilt in ensuring that all has been done, but unfortunately, patients can linger needlessly in this strange environment.

Denny: Tested but Not Treated

Denny was successful and well known in his community for his public service and political work. In his sixties, he'd been my patient for several years. His lymphoma was worsening. His kidneys were failing, and he was losing weight. Bitter and upset, he decided to go to a large center out of state. Once he arrived there, Denny had three bone marrow biopsies in a week in a half. He endured one test after another.

Not one of those tests provided him any hope or comfort. He died on dialysis three months later, while on a ventilator in an ICU out of state.

Although no one could have saved his life at that point, I know his last days could have been made more comfortable.

WHEN A LARGE CENTER IS THE WISE CHOICE

The large centers are equipped to handle some situations your local oncologist cannot. In many cases, they are your best treatment option.

WHEN SHOULD YOU GO?

- When the center has a specific piece of equipment you need for treatment.
- When your type of cancer requires coordination among many surgeons and specialists with specific technical expertise.
- When the clinic has years of experience developing treatments for a specific, rare cancer.
- When you feel a specific center or physician would be helpful to you.
- When the research program at the large center has a treatment option unavailable elsewhere.

- When you need reassurance that the treatment you are receiving closer to home is best.

Jill: Numerous Surgeons Needed

Jill, a 28-year-old teacher in a small community, was diagnosed with cervical cancer. At that time, the cancer was too far advanced for her to have surgery to remove it—her treatment was going to involve reconstructing her female organs. That meant she needed a gynecologic surgeon, a bowel surgeon, a urologist, a plastic surgeon for reconstructing her vagina, and a radiation therapist at the time her abdomen was opened. It's difficult to get all of those doctors in the same room at the same time even at a large center. Anywhere else, it's close to impossible. In Jill's case, the large center was the right choice.

WHAT TO BRING WHEN YOU GO

If you and your doctor decide that the large cancer center is for you, what next?

In addition to a friend or family member, you should also bring the following with you.

- Multiple copies of an updated, concise summary of your case written by your physician for this purpose. It's useful if this summary includes a specific question your doctor wants addressed.
- CD copies (not originals) of all of your relevant X-ray images, including important CT and PET scans and MRIs.
- Your local oncologist's contact information and the way he prefers to be reached.
- Copies of business cards for all your physicians.
- Contact information for your insurance company, particularly those individuals in charge of preapproving treatment.
- A current list of all your medications and allergies.
- Your pathology slides.
- A lot of patience.

You want your visit to be worthwhile. It's important to transmit information in a timely way that will help avoid confusion, redundancy, and useless trips — and get you the best care.

BEST OF BOTH WORLDS

Do you choose the big cancer center or your local oncologist? It's only an either/or situation if you have the wrong doctor on either side. For unusual tumors that your oncologist doesn't see every day, it makes sense to go to a center. You don't necessarily have to be treated at that center, however. The center doctors' advice means more if they're able to collaborate more with your community oncologist, and they often are.

Carmen: Cooperative Treatment Worked Well

Carmen, a 35-year-old woman, came to see me complaining of vague abdominal pain, flushing, and hot flashes. Surgery found an endocrine tumor in her pancreas. Results of a second surgery at a large cancer center revealed that the tumor had spread to several different areas. They couldn't remove it all and offered Carmen chemotherapy.

She started it at the cancer center, and we continued her treatment locally when Carmen returned home. As she improved, she traveled back and forth between the center and our clinic. Carmen's treatment is now complete, and she is doing great. She went to the large center, got a plan of care, and has done well since then. She also made sure that she had her local oncologist nearby.

COOPERATION AND COORDINATION

A word to the wise: If a center demands that you *only* be treated there, ask for their motives. You need to understand the reasons why they feel strongly about how your care is handled. By asking the right questions, you'll be able to understand the attitude of the cancer center and your comfort level in complying with their suggestions.

Here's a list of questions you should ask:

- Does the center have hands-on experience treating patients with the same tumor or specialize in *only* that type of tumor?
- Is there a patient with the same type of tumor who's done well on this treatment? If so, can they make arrangements for you to talk with this patient? Most patients are willing to share information.
- Are they willing to collaborate with your local oncologist?
- Are they willing to advocate for you within the system?
- Will they be available?

Be aware that not every local oncologist will be willing to work with you if you've gone to a big center. This is important, because you may want to choose this person carefully. You need to know you have the support of your local doctor and that, if circumstances warrant it, he will actually pick up the phone or write a letter for you.

Be assured that there are many local oncologists who will be there for their patients, regardless of the care sought or where they seek it. Their concern, ultimately, is the patient's welfare, not their egos. Don't be intimidated. It is in your best interest that you should be the priority, not someone's feelings. A good oncologist will talk to whomever will be in charge of your care and find out what you're actually getting into. Are you going to have to do this forever? Is there a drug available that may work for you now? They'll ask these questions for you.

Rebecca: Too Late for Consultations

Rebecca had allowed us to treat her metastatic breast cancer for many years. She had been through surgery, radiation, hormone therapy, and a plethora of chemotherapy treatments. While they had been helpful over the years, her condition had gradually weakened, and the tumor had grown increasingly resistant. She was hospitalized more and more in the last several months. Her husband had been very attentive and was at every appointment. Her children, some of whom were from a distance away, hadn't been to many visits. When her family physician, her oncologist, and her husband recommended comfort measures and hospice, she agreed.

Even though she was bedridden, her sister disagreed and began a discussion to have her transferred to a large cancer center several states away. She had wanted to ensure that all had been done to help her. Rebecca wasn't able to walk; she was essentially bedridden and was developing liver and kidney failure.

After a long discussion, her sister agreed to her comfort measures plans. Her wish for a consultation grew out of a sincere desire to ensure that her sister had explored all possible options for treatment. She had not kept up with Rebecca's illness during her regular visits and hadn't asked earlier for a consultation when her sister's condition was better. At this time, late in her course, a consultation at the major cancer center would have only served to reassure them that all possible options had been considered, while putting Rebecca through quite a bit of inconvenience at a very difficult time of her life.

QUESTIONS TO ASK

If you've already evaluated your doctor as someone who is compassionate and wants to do his best, but may be out of his league in terms of knowledge or expertise, be honest about your concerns. Ask, "Would you still help me if I get an opinion at the ABC Clinic?" If the answer is negative, consider finding another oncologist.

Another question to ask is, "If I've had my first several treatments at a cancer center, and I do okay, will you still treat me here?"

Ideally, what you want is for your local oncologist and the person from the big cancer center working together in a three-point relationship that is cooperative, not antagonistic. If either refuses to work with the other, choose another doctor.

EMPOWER YOURSELF

1. Don't go to a major cancer center by yourself. Consult your local oncologist before you do anything else.
2. Unless your oncologist knows of a specific study to get you into, it may be preferable to begin treatment locally first. Although doing so will make you ineligible for a clinical study, delaying treatment by as little as a week can have potentially life-threatening implications.

3. Maintain a strong medical and personal support group in your hometown. This will give you great peace of mind.
4. Make sure the expectations are clear on the treatment you're getting, especially when you're considering Phase I studies.

WHAT'S NEXT

Insurance can be your best friend—or worst enemy—when navigating the cancer system. If your insurance coverage isn't ideal, you need to learn what to do about it, as well as where to find help when you must challenge insurance decisions.

Chapter 7

Insurance Angles
Making the System Work for You

In a utopian world, everyone would have perfect health coverage and the best treatment possible. Reality is far different. Problems happen. You may lose coverage midway through your illness. Bills mount up, and credit cards get maxed out. Collections notices arrive with no paycheck. Or worse yet, you may find yourself uninsured and suddenly disabled and diagnosed with an advanced cancer. Finding care quickly with no coverage is difficult, but not impossible. However, this chapter will give you the basics to understand a system that has been made deliberately complex. Of course, the more convoluted the system, the harder it is for ill patients to navigate to get their care. Luckily there are many ways to help, including appropriate government programs.

WHY INSURANCE?

Whether or not you like the idea of insurance, it's essential. It tells your oncologist several key things about you. It shows that you are a responsible member of the community. It also tells the doctor that you will be able to pay. Further, it protects you from unmonitored oncologists who might stray from good cancer care.

Your doctor may be worried that uninsured patients are more likely to sue. Remember that your oncologist is under no obligation to care for you. You are asking for his expertise.

Thomas: No Care for Medicare Patient

Thomas, an 85-year-old World War II veteran who witnessed the atom bomb blast at Bikini Island, had survived three cancers. He has Medicare, a supplemental Medicare policy, and a Medicare D plan. Medicare D plans are the prescription drug plans of Medicare. He decided to move to a large city to be near his children, but he wasn't able to find a physician there who accepted Medicare. Even though Tom had Medicare, however, doesn't mean that he could find a physician to accept him. And if he could find a benevolent oncologist, he might still not be able to assemble an entire team—radiologist, nursing home, rehab center, neurosurgeon, and urologist—whose members would be willing to take him on as a patient. Tom decided to remain at home, although distant from his children, chiefly for this reason.

Payment problems can be another obstacle if you are uninsured. It is not the doctor's responsibility to worry about where the thousands of dollars to treat you will be found. It is your responsibility. If you don't have insurance, you will need to personally negotiate for each service, drug, and scan. Also, if you have no insurance and self pay, you have no bargaining power and no say in what your actual fees are. In addition to paying an exorbitant amount, you'd end up spending 30-50 percent *more* than any insurance company would have paid.

Expensive boutique offices in large cities do exist that accept private pay patients who pay cash. Many visit these clinics from another country for the sole purpose of receiving their treatments. The monthly payments for these services may be as high as $80,000. Only a handful of patients a day can afford these rates.

INSURANCE BASICS

It is no surprise that the people who have the best coverage sometimes get priority in being accepted first as patients. Appointments are made sooner. Having insurance reassures an oncologist both that he will be able to find appropriate care for you and that he will get paid for these services. But it's not that simple. There are many details. If you don't play your cards right, you can find yourself out of luck with no care even though you have good insurance. It is true that when you have no insurance coverage you'll need to work harder and think fast to get care. But it is possible to get coverage. This is the time to let your family and friends help you. You may want to engage the help of a spouse, sibling, or friend.

You will learn more about Medicare and Medicaid later in this chapter. These are extraordinarily complicated government programs even when you aren't sick. Forms, appeals, denials, and dismissal letters can be overwhelming. Government programs are very rigid and are often administered in a stale bureaucratic and inhumane manner. Offices that close early for lunch (or yet another federal holiday), delays due to unfilled positions, and bureaucratic inertia all combine to make government programs frustrating.

INSURANCE AND EMPLOYERS

Most of us feel resigned to the insurance assigned to us by our employers. But your insurance is not static, it is fluid. It changes often. Having and keeping good health care coverage is an important first step to getting the best care. And it is really possible to get insurance coverage after you are diagnosed with cancer. Flexibility and portability are most important. You want the option to keep your insurance throughout your illness. It is also important to have the least restrictive coverage that doesn't limit your oncologist's choices for your treatment.

There is no Web site you can go to that tells you which insurance company allows your physician the most flexibility in coverage and good reimbursements. Because of rising health care costs, employer groups are routinely lured into changing to carriers that cut corners or limit access to providers. The employers themselves often don't appreciate how limiting the policy they purchased is. They didn't know that the new coverage makes you drive 45 minutes out of your way each time you need blood work. All that the employer often knows is how much money the company is saving each year with the new policy. If the new insurance company delayed the business owner's chemotherapy by a month though, he'd be upset also.

The insurance product paid for by your employer applies to everyone in the group. This fact may allow you to lobby your employer and change to insurance with better coverage when appropriate. With enough feedback from you, the employee, and others, gradual change for the better can occur. With enough complaints, the state office regulating the insurer may also act.

KNOW YOUR INSURANCE

Soon after diagnosis, try to spend some time with your employer's personnel department so that you better understand your policy. All policies have innumerable nuances and fine print. In which calendar year were the services rendered? Did you get a referral? Was the provider in network or out of network? You should know as many of the details as possible. Does your medical insurance consider paying for dental care to treat oral complications of your radiation treatments? Does your cancer policy consider myelodysplastic disorders as cancers or not? (They are.) Myelodysplastic disorders are blood disorders that may be considered preleukemic. Can you use a spouse's redundant policy also?

WHY CODING MATTERS

Coding is how your hospital or physician charges the insurance company for each specific treatment that is done. The coders tell the insurance company how many doses of treatment are given, on which day they were done, and for what specific reason. Coding explains why your doctor doesn't want to take off both skin lesions at once. If the dermatologist removes two on the same day, he gets paid a full fee for the first lesion and half for the second. Coding is why your doctor rarely calls you back himself. Your attorney gets paid for phone consultations. Your doctor does not. Although Medicare has a code to charge for telephone visits, little or nothing is paid, so no calls happen.

HOW TO KEEP YOUR INSURANCE

If you have a spouse who is employed and has insurance that covers the family, consider yourself lucky. Tragic consequences occur when the only jobholder in the family contracts cancer. If you lose your job and are unable to secure another, you may want to pay to keep your current employer-sponsored insurance. While the cost may seem substantial, it will always be better than being uninsured. Laws exist that permit the employee to pay for health insurance for eighteen months. (Unfortunately this is six months short of the twenty four months that it may take Medicare disability to kick in). Other avenues to stay insured, if you lose your job and current policy, include having your spouse move to a job with better coverage. Your preexisting conditions may be covered when your spouse starts a new job with group health insurance.

UNDERSTAND YOUR BILLS

Even the most savvy physicians and accountants have trouble with their medical bills. They are a nightmare. It is very confusing to try to understand how much you actually owe. Have someone in the business office of the medical center or clinic where you are being treated explain them to you face to face. Repeatedly. You may have to return regularly to the office as your account changes.

Try to get the name of a specific person assigned to your case. Get the direct phone number for that individual. Ask to speak to a supervisor if this person appears unknowledgeable or if there is a disagreement. Be firm but mannerly. Try not to be confrontational. Developing a positive relationship with this office is essential.

STAY ON TOP OF YOUR BILLS.

Bills are complicated. Delays in filing occur. Physician's offices make mistakes. Insurance companies make mistakes, and you may make mistakes. Don't assume that bills are correct. Often they are not. Normally it takes several months for them to be reconciled. The amount charged by the physician is rarely paid in full. Discounts (called write offs) of varying amounts are taken off the bill by the insurer, depending on the previously accepted arrangements. You need to be aware of the specific charges for which you are responsible. Trying to figure out the remaining amount owed is sometimes very challenging.

PAY YOUR BILLS

It is important to keep your account current. Physician offices and hospitals are increasingly running on tighter and tighter margins. As such, they are under pressure to make the most of the balance owed to them. When you are tardy in your payments, you give the health care facility a good reason to dismiss you. Remember, you need their care. Keeping your records in good graces is very important. Many families become caught between trying to decide what is worse: having their account sent to a collection agency or adding even more debt to their credit card account. Since many clinics, offices, and hospitals don't charge interest on accounts, it pays to do your best to work within their business accounts system.

If you have spectacular insurance but don't pay your copays and deductibles, you could lose your doctor. In your household record keeping, you should assume that you will be paying the full amount of your deductible each year. This needs to go as a line in your monthly household budget. Any amount you don't end up paying is gravy. Pay these bills before you pay the cable TV bill. Your health is more important.

DON'T GET SENT TO COLLECTIONS

It is critical to stay out of collections. This is the kiss of death. Once your account goes to collections, you develop an unfavorable reputation. With the cost of cancer care and higher copays and deductibles, however, avoiding collections is hard for most people. Tactics to avoid having your account sent to collections are many. Here are some tips.

One avenue is to make payment arrangement ahead of time with the clinic's business offices. If you do this, you may want to get it in writing. A verbal arrangement with a midlevel manager may not be binding. Consider paying the most important offices first. Not-for-profit hospital systems may allow you more leeway with your account. These types of facilities may also have foundations to help pay some of your account.

Collection policies may and do change frequently. You may also want to contest any part of your bill you think is debatable. Applying for aid from various community and benevolent groups may also keep part of your bill from being seen as delinquent. Other means include applying for disability through federal and state programs (see the Resources section at the end of the book).

APPEAL ALL INSURANCE PAYMENT DENIALS

Recruit the help of your oncologist's office to appeal when the insurance company denies your claim. He will know the specific clinical situation that best justifies payment. The oncologist is responsible for documenting this in his notes. The pharmaceutical company responsible for the drug involved may also help by directing your oncologist toward research information showing positive studies that document a treatment to be useful. Insurance companies are also more likely to pay when they hear that other insurers are also currently paying for similar cancer treatment situations.

PRIVATE INSURANCE PROGRAMS

Commercial health insurance is expected among working-age families. As insurance becomes more expensive, this expectation becomes less common. Increasingly much of the cost of this coverage has been forced on to you, the consumer. It may be little consolation, but improvements in drugs, health care, and technology are partly responsible for the increased expenses. While employer-sponsored programs are the norm for many, millions don't fall into this lucky group. Still, commercial insurance is usually a good deal. Many different types of programs, including PPOs and HMOs, exist from which to choose. However, problems can occur regardless of which type of coverage you have.

INSURANCE PROBLEMS

The first problem to avoid is a lapse. A break in your insurance is very bad. You don't want a lapse in your coverage. If you have insurance from company A, try very hard to avoid going uninsured for several months. All of your medical problems will essentially become preexisting when you do regain insurance. Preexisting conditions are conditions that were present before and as such may be excluded

The hyperattentive monitors "helping" organize and "manage" your care can also present a problem. These well-intentioned nurses who perform this service are often assigned to protect the insurance company's agenda at your expense. Ask your oncologist if their help is needed before signing on with them. If they call and offer to help, don't automatically acquiesce and agree to their services.

Other insurance problems that may arise include tardiness in approving second- and third- line drugs for off-label treatments. Little motivation exists for insurance companies to speedily approve off-label drugs. While these treatments may truly be in your best interest, the ambiguities involved in approving drugs in the research and approval pipeline can cause unfortunate delays.

Rachael: Aggressive Treatment Denied

Rachael is a 50-year-old government employee with commercial insurance. When her breast cancer spread to a single liver area, her oncologist gave her chemotherapy. After several months, the lesion had improved incompletely. Her oncologist recommended surgical evaluation. However, the site of the cancer was too difficult for the surgeon to access safely. It was tucked up in the dome of the liver, under the diaphragm. Luckily, this resourceful surgeon was able to eradicate the cancer with a special probe. However, her insurance failed to see the wisdom of this approach and failed to pay for the surgery. After some negotiation, the hospital and physician wrote off the remainder of her bill.

It may take months or longer to aggressively pursue getting something paid for, and your insurance company may still deny it. If this happens, you can always appeal to the physician himself.

PREAPPROVAL

Assume that each treatment, consultation, and scan ordered for your cancer treatment will need to be preapproved by your insurer. Usually this is straightforward when standard guidelines are being followed. You can't assume, however, that the preapproval letter will be honored when the bill is submitted. Preapproved means that the insurance company agrees that the treatment is indicated. At times, a treatment may be preapproved but the treatment asked for may not be covered by your policy. Try to ask specifically if the preapproval letter obligates the insurer to pay.

Other insurance and payment problems occur in several instances. These include when your oncologist considers a treatment for a cancer that does not have a standard treatment. This unfortunately occurs more often in rare cancers where research is not as current. For those who have them, it may not be known whether many currently available drugs will help. This is because few patients are able to enroll in clinical trials. You may also run into problems when a treatment is thought to be incompletely studied or is not standard. Guidelines are appropriate and useful for most situations, but it is acceptable to consider off-label treatments when the standard ones fail.

If there is incomplete data, you may need to seek out clinical trials. Although they are always an option, they may be difficult to find and access. Another fine point that can lead to disappointment is when the treatment is preapproved (meaning that the insurer thinks that the treatment is a good idea), but it is not a covered service. This means that you have a policy that doesn't cover it. Perhaps your policy doesn't cover reconstructive surgery or mental health care. You need to ask both questions. Is it approved and is it a covered service?

OUTSIDE CONSULTANTS

Another problem common to many insurance programs is when you select an oncologist who is not on the list of preferred providers. One option is for you to offer to pay out of pocket for consultations with the outside oncologist. To keep your expenses low, you might consider receiving your treatment from the in-house preferred oncologist. You could still see the outside oncologist occasionally for strategic planning. On rare occasions you may even find it possible to ask the outside oncologist and his office to consider becoming a preferred provider.

Private insurers can also have a more human side and are able to listen to the pleas of you and your oncologist. The oncologist can call the medical director directly and appeal a denial. This is in contrast to the hard and fast bureaucratic approach required of most government programs.

PRESCRIPTION COVERAGE

When choosing prescription coverage, try to avoid plans that require higher fees for nongeneric or brand-name drugs. You need coverage for your doctor to treat you with medications you need. Generics may work fine for uncomplicated hypertension diabetes or diabetes treatment, but for cancer, there are rarely replacements for many of the latest drugs. Newer drugs could be on patent for many years.

A scary kind of denial can occur when you have prescriptions for only generics. You are financially motivated to use the generic treatment the insurance is covering. The VA system often morphs into generic treatment only. Often patients will insist on taking the less expensive but substandard treatment. Patients delay or refuse the expensive but better treatment so as to limit the out-of-pocket expenses.

Joe: Only Generics

Joe was a respiratory therapist with lung cancer, who could benefit from oral chemotherapy. Unfortunately the pills cost more than his monthly salary. His insurance wouldn't cover any brand name drugs. The programs that might be able to assist in the payment of his prescription drugs wouldn't help because he had a form of prescription coverage and because he was above the income limits.

"We don't need the new drugs," he told me. "Good old generics work just as well." They don't.

Generic drugs to treat most common cancers are not available. But the patient in the sidebar above is in a financial trap that could cost his life. All you're saying when you ask for generics is that you don't want the new technology; you'll take the older stuff.

The worst plans are those that require you to pay high percentage co-pays for nongeneric prescriptions. Plans where you pay 50 percent of prescription drugs are terrible. Limited compassionate assistance is available for copays. So, if you have a nest egg or a good income, you pay the 50 percent copays. For a $3,000-per-month drug, this could be a prohibitive $1,500 per month. You might be tempted to forgo such treatments rather than spend that much out of pocket.

SPECIALTY PHARMACIES

These pharmacies deal only with superexpensive oral drugs. They specialize in medications normally costing approximately $3,000 per month. You receive the drugs by mail. The companies and their representatives market themselves to your oncologist and can be of critical help to you. They know you won't be able to pay a high out-of-pocket expense each month. Pharmaceutical companies delegate their reimbursement help to outside companies that work with these specialist pharmacies. Together they look at all possibilities of help (including disease-specific foundations, veterans and state programs, and drug company programs) to find a way to get you the drugs you need.

Local nonprofit foundations may exist to help patients defer expenses. These and other foundations might pay costs related to nausea medication or drugs to strengthen your bones, as well as for a specific kind of cancer. Sometimes local cancer societies also have programs to help.

MEDICARE AND MEDICAID PROGRAMS

Medicare applies to all patients over the age of 65 and to those who have been disabled. You need to be disabled for two years and have paid into the social security system to be eligible for Medicare under these criteria. Several important caveats apply to you when you have Medicare. The first is that Medicare only pays 80 percent of hospital and outpatient bills. It rarely pays the entire amount charged. Almost always there is a write-off where Medicare disallows a substantial portion of the charge. Hospitals and physician offices expect reduced payments. After Medicare decides how much of the charge is allowed, it pays 80 percent, and you are responsible for the remaining 20 percent.

If your doctor or hospital did not ask you to sign a waiver to agree to pay for off-label treatments before receiving care, they cannot charge you for a treatment if Medicare denies paying for it. If Medicare doesn't pay its 80 percent, then your supplemental will not pay anything. Most people think that their coinsurance will cover the treatments that Medicare denies. Not so. The supplemental insurance decides nothing; they pay only the 20 percent that Medicare doesn't pay. If Medicare denies payment, so do they.

Medicare Part A pays for inpatient services. **Part B** pays for outpatient services. Medicare D programs pay for prescriptions. With a few exceptions, only part D plans pay for prescriptions, not part A or B. Part D plans can be purchased each year. If you don't have a part D prescription plan, you run the risk of not being able to afford crucial drugs. Most cancer-related drugs are unaffordable for the average family. In addition to oral chemotherapy agents, many other expensive prescriptions, such as nausea drugs, antibiotics, and pain medications, can drive up the monthly cost. By limiting your coverage, you restrict your own treatment options substantially. Laws and regulations regarding Medicare payments change yearly and always at the last minute.

Cancer treatment is so expensive that almost nobody can afford to pay the copays remaining after Medicare pays its 80 percent. A common flaw is assuming that you can afford this 20 percent copay. Budgeting based on last year's expenses is similar to driving a car looking out of the back and not the front window. You are only eligible to purchase a Medicare supplemental policy for a very short window of time around your retirement age, but you should buy them. Many people aren't aware of these limitations to Medicare supplemental policies, but you can learn about the timing of signing up for them from the social security agency and local senior citizen support organizations. After that, you are out of luck. Your only option will be to try to apply for other government programs such as Medicaid when your assets are spent.

Medicare supplemental policies are a great bargain. It is almost impossible to receive serious cancer treatment without one. Without such a policy, there is tremendous heartache. You may find yourself stopping treatment for financial, not medical, reasons. An unmarried person could spend nearly all of his or her assets and then qualify to apply for government assistance. It is unusual for a married person to spend nearly all of the family's remaining financial assets and leave the other spouse impoverished. When placed in this awful position, couples often make the difficult decision to limit treatment. The sad part is that much of this is preventable with good planning. By being flexible and open to addressing financial concerns, you can avoid many of these pitfalls.

As previously mentioned, take out a supplemental policy while you are eligible. If you don't have such a policy and are too old to purchase one, consider the following options. You and your spouse could consider a division of assets. This is where the family assets are divided in two. Yours are spent on your health care. The remainder can stay with your survivor. This occurs frequently when one spouse needs to go into a nursing home. If you wish to give assets to your heirs, this will need to be done several years earlier. Otherwise, those assets are still considered yours. A division of assets, however, can be done at any time.

Medicare D

Medicare D plans cover prescription medications. In these unnecessarily complicated plans, the patient pays all costs of an initial $250 deductible. This is followed by the "D" plan paying the costs of the drugs up to an amount of approximately $2700. If you have prescription drug costs above this, you may find yourself in the unfortunate "donut hole." This is where you pay the entire costs of the next $1200 of drug expenses. After this, the "D" plan resumes coverage of 95 percent of remaining expenses.

The real life effect of the donut hole is that many patients taking long-term drugs, such as oral medication to prevent breast cancer from returning, often unfortunately decide to not fill the prescription during the last several months of the year. For those patients who need to take drugs costing $3000 per month or more, the donut hole comes during the first month. In addition the 5 percent of catastrophic costs add up quickly.

AGEISM

Many people nearing the age of 65 view Medicare as a free government oasis in a desert of high-priced insurance. Once they're on the Medicare plan, many discover it's not what it appeared from a distance. Instead, they realize that they have made a one-way trip into the world of "Healthcare for the Old."

For example, at the age of 55, Mrs. Jones is told to return regularly for cholesterol checks. At the age of 72, despite having many complex problems, she doesn't get a return appointment scheduled. She's simply told to return when she's sick. The 35-year-old weekend athlete with a mild shoulder injury, however, might get an appointment in 48 hours. Conversely, the 80-year-old with a hip injury threatening his ability to live independently is told that the next available appointment is two or three months down the road. These subtleties exist because of the inequity between Medicare and the private insurance system.

It is possible, and at times even advantageous, to try to continue to use private insurance as your primary coverage even after you reach the age of 65. At the very least, it's a good idea to have a Medicare supplement policy. Also don't plan your insurance based on what your needs were last year; plan ahead for any eventuality.

The way treatment options are presented and encouraged may depend on your age and not on your health. I recently saw a patient, age 67, who was told by a doctor that he was "too old" to be treated for his cancer. Perhaps the doctor was having a bad day, or perhaps the patient looked ill when examined. Or maybe the patient was just too "Medicared" to be treated. His was not a difficult cancer, and he is doing well since we started treating him.

MEDICARE: SAME CANCER, DIFFERENT STATE, DIFFERENT COVERAGE

If you have lymphoma and live in Florida, is the disease any different than in Kansas? It is to Medicare—and to the one physician who gets to decide what the coverage will be in your state. That's right. As inconsistent as that sounds, it's true. Medicare doesn't have a national policy for what it pays for. While most treatments follow standard protocol, in certain situations, your physician will need some flexibility in your treatment.

For example, Medicare regional medical directors enjoy leeway in deciding whether to pay for certain chemotherapy drugs. One way to learn about which chemotherapy drugs may be useful for specific cancers is when an agent is listed in an approved source known as a compendia. Previously, when a chemotherapy drug was listed in one of the several compendia, Medicare reimbursement was automatic. Regional differences in payment trends have occurred because some administrators interpret this compendia listing as only a guideline—not a requirement. Lung cancer patients in one state may be able to have a particular biologic drug that was initially approved and commercially available to treat another cancer paid for by Medicare, while patients in other states are not. This flexibility differs from state to state, depending on the medical administrator, who may or may not be an oncologist.

Medicare is not insurance. It is a government program. It is not subject to market forces. If you are a private business owner and are unsatisfied with one insurance company, you can effect real change by voting with your feet and moving your insurance to another company. Not so with Medicare. Layers on layers of bureaucracy, elected officials, and government forms keep this type of feedback from affecting those whose service is poor. Physician providers are subject to both civil and criminal penalties for violations. Unlike insurance companies, such as Blue Cross, Medicare does not preauthorize any treatment but, instead, gives some idea as to which treatments will be covered. Even when Medicare has paid for a particular treatment, that doesn't mean that the issue is final. Medicare can and does audit its payments. Just because they paid for a certain service doesn't mean that they can't come back and change their mind later and reclaim payments.

MEDICAID

Medicaid is a federally mandated and state administered health care program for the poor. An advanced cancer may also make you eligible for disability. Once you've had disability and Medicaid for two years, you might get Medicare if you have worked and paid into social security for a long enough time. After you're 65 years old, you're no longer disabled in the eyes of the government. Instead, you receive Social Security. Essentially, disabled people are just getting their Social Security check early. If you have cancer at any age and are uninsured, apply for Medicaid at once, as it may be retroactive to the date of application. If you haven't worked for enough months and paid into the social security system, you may not be eligible for disability.

It is important to wait to apply for Medicaid disability benefits when you are not working. If you are, you are likely not eligible. A different deductible for each person is also calculated called a spend down. This means subtracting $495 from your monthly income. In this way, the deductible is based on your income. It is recalculated every six months.

NO INSURANCE?

If you have no insurance coverage and have a rapidly worsening condition, the first step is to consider going to the emergency room. They have the resources to rapidly evaluate and triage you. The emergency room physician will consult by phone with various specialist physicians if needed. After that, a decision will be made about whether or not you need to be admitted.

Here are some creative yet legal ways patients have dealt with the problem of no insurance.

SPOUSE CHANGES JOBS

A patient is an artist married to a man who has his own auto repair shop. Neither thought health care coverage was important, and now she has been diagnosed with breast cancer. They have assets, but no coverage. Although the husband enjoyed working for himself, the priority became his wife's illness and how to get the best coverage. He went to work for a large automobile dealership with a good group plan.

PATIENT CHANGES JOBS

If you're capable of working, you might consider leaving your current job for one with health insurance. Just because you have cancer and are working for one employer doesn't mean you can't go to another employer with better insurance.

PATIENT PURCHASES HIGH-RISK INSURANCE

You might also get insurance through the state-sponsored high-risk insurance pools for the uninsured. These pools are targeted to patients denied health coverage because they are considered a high risk to insurers. The programs charge premiums, which are fees you have to pay. There may also be copayments and deductibles which means you are responsible for part of the fee. Although the premiums are higher than those for standard insurance, they are also capped or have a life-time spending limit.

The state-sponsored programs often have waiting periods for preexisting conditions and limits on enrollment. For example, you may remain without insurance coverage for the preexisting conditions for the first 90 days. For this time period, you may be forced to pay out of pocket or look for other avenues to get you care. But during this time, don't wait to see your oncologist, who can help you decide what the best short-term plan is. Sometimes it is better to compromise slightly on the best available treatment than to get no treatment at all. Patients may use them only until they qualify for another program. If you are eligible for Medicare or Medicaid, you will not qualify. You will also need to be a state resident for a set number of months to be eligible.

At this writing, state-sponsored programs exist in Alabama, Alaska, Arkansas, California, Colorado, Florida, Illinois, Indiana, Iowa, Kansas, Kentucky, Louisiana, Maryland, Minnesota, Mississippi, Missouri, Montana, Nebraska, New Hampshire, New Mexico, North Dakota, Oklahoma, Oregon, South Carolina, South Dakota, Tennessee, Texas, Utah, Washington State, Utah, Washington, Wisconsin, and Wyoming. (See the Resources section.)

PATIENT GETS MEDICAID OR MEDICARE

It isn't that difficult to eventually get Medicaid after being diagnosed with advanced cancer. More challenging is trying to find a team of physicians to care for you if Medicaid is your only coverage. Single specialty clinics or individual providers may not be able to help the Medicaid patient as much as a larger clinics or health care systems.

DISABILITY COVERAGE

It helps to have private disability coverage that's as flexible and generous as it can be. Also if you have no emergency fund and your need to wait for six months for disability to kicks in, you might as well have no disability coverage. Read your disability plan. Understand what it covers and run through a rainy-day scenario with your family the way you would run through a fire emergency plan. Ask questions like, "What would we do if Dad was disabled? How would we make our expenses?" Motivated and flexible employers may be able to help by advancing future pay.

Dale: No Disability Plan Limits Options

Dale is in his late forties and, until he got lymphoma, he was able to handle a strenuous job of building boats. As the disease progressed, he was getting tired, worn out, and weak. He had nothing in savings to fall back on, and the only disability he had was Social Security, which would not cover him unless he was unable to work at all. If he stops working now, his job would not pay him nor would he get any money from disability for six to nine months. He can't afford to do that.

This lack of preparation can lead to a financial indication for prematurely stopping treatment.

LONG-TERM CARE CONSIDERATIONS

It is not unusual for cancer patients to occasionally benefit from a brief stay in a nursing home, especially at the beginning or end of their treatment. Sometimes assistance in the home is also needed. Nursing home expenses can add up rapidly, thus worsening the stress on the patient and family.

Optimally, a flexible long-term health care insurance plan is able to pay for both nursing home care and long-term home care. If not, then in some situations, the couple's assets are divided in half. In this division of assets the ill person's half is spent on the nursing home or other medical expenses, while the well person's half remains with him or her. When the patient's assets are exhausted, Medicaid pays.

EMPOWER YOURSELF

Think of insurance as an obstacle course. The more challenges you give your doctor, the more difficult it is for him to run the race with you. Don't put ten layers of bureaucracy between your doctor and your coverage.

WHAT'S NEXT

Chemotherapy has a bad reputation, and much of it is unearned. In the next chapter, we're going to look at the most common chemotherapy myths and the way selection of chemotherapy drugs is sometimes based, not on your needs, but on profit.

Chapter 8

Chemotherapy, Radiation, Surgery
Innovations, Promises, and Pitfalls

You've heard that cancer treatments worsen your quality of life, but the opposite can often be true as well. Years ago, early treatments for cancer were viewed with enthusiasm and promise, but in reality, they had poorly treatable side effects that limited their usefulness. The effectiveness of treatments today almost uniformly exceeds patients' expectations. Don't allow legends and myths to keep you from reaching the best outcome possible.

Patients usually expect to require only one of the following therapies: chemotherapy, radiation, or surgery. Not so. Today's cancer treatments achieve better results by employing a combination of two or three therapies. Chemotherapy is often combined with radiation. Surgery is often followed by radiation. Chemotherapy may be used first to shrink the tumor and then surgery or radiation.

A patient's first step should be to listen to a serious discussion of the various cancer treatment options; this discussion can have a monumental impact on treatment. As a result of vivid memories of loved ones who have suffered through cancer and its treatment, patients sometimes refuse treatment and succumb to potentially treatable conditions. They died without *even listening* to treatment options. It is essential that you are able to carefully listen, ask appropriate questions, and then make informed decisions. By knowing the latest information, you can greatly improve your chances of successful treatment, with a good quality of life. It is important that you understand some general information about the various ways that cancer is treated.

Cancers have long been dread diseases with imminent and painful death expected. Initially, years ago, oncologists used radical (and sometimes overly toxic) chemotherapy and radiation treatments that they expected you to tolerate for even the smallest of benefits. Useful drugs that effectively limit side effects are mostly a development of the last several years. For many patients, remembering what made grandpa sick many years ago becomes jumbled in a mix of drug or radiation side effects or symptoms of the cancer itself. Many patients have understandably low expectations.

Lately, newer cancer treatments have been developed that are more easily tolerated and have far more manageable side effects. New therapies can be built on the limited successes of the pioneering initial treatments. Through these methods, doctors have begun to incrementally understand how to improve chances of success. By the time a patient is engaged in the cancer treatment process, these myriad advances found throughout all aspects of cancer treatment combine to make it a much more tolerable and effective journey.

You may hear about various therapies through your friends who have cancer. Listening to a bewildering number of claims about chemotherapy and radiation can confuse and scare you. Rarely does this kind of exchange reassure a patient. Some experiences are frightening, while others are overly optimistic. In this chapter, you will learn when each of these treatments might be useful. Simply understanding the timing or sequencing of the treatments can be very important, even life saving.

For example, when a lung cancer is correctly staged as an advanced stage III in the chest only, your treatment could appropriately involve primarily radiation or surgery. Whatever choice is made, it is important to understand the rationale that justifies a physician's recommendation. For example, the physician might find it difficult to resign the patient at a young age to an incurable stage IV cancer. In a bout of optimism, he wrongly assumes the cancer to be only in the chest. He may suggest aggressive surgical or radiation treatment for stage III lung cancer. Unfortunately, this surgery or radiation may be dangerous in that it ignores treatment for other sites of the cancer. The lung cancer found involving the chest is quickly and expertly eradicated, but as the chest heals, quietly and quickly, the cancer grows in other areas, such as the adrenal glands, liver, brain, or spine. All of these are areas to which lung cancer can spread. The bone scan was, therefore, wrong. The intensive local therapy of surgery or radiation therapy that was useful and appropriate for stage III delayed the initiation of treatments that could target all areas of the cancer. This surgery or radiation is a incomplete if a stage is really a more advanced stage IV. Both the patient and the physician need to be honest with themselves so that the patient can get the best treatment.

SURGERY

Surgery is the oldest and most established method used to treat cancer. Surgeons who have developed pioneering procedures can be found occupying prestigious positions at major universities. These groundbreaking methods can help you and others benefit from new organ-sparing techniques. Other new techniques include limited exposure laparoscopic surgery, which speeds recovery time. Still other techniques allow a surgeon to more aggressively remove extensive tumors. You might also have heard friends marvel at the accomplishments of reconstructive surgeons. It is a testament to the importance of surgery that despite many years of other cancer treatment advances, surgery still holds the major role in the treatment of many tumors.

A family might spend hours in waiting rooms expecting to hear a weary surgeon's definitive words, "I got it all." There was a capsule around the tumor. It was isolated. *I got it all.* Yes, this is good news. But is it all you need to know? No.

Patients quickly form close bonds with their surgeons. You have trusted your body, your cancer, and your life to this person, and she or he wants to help. Surgeons naturally want to reassure you that their handiwork was successful. Yes, the pain, the suffering, the inconvenience was worth it. You're okay.

You want a confident surgeon who doesn't doubt himself. Operating on cancer patients can be trying for the ego, however. Many times, patients have complications or the tumor recurs. At times, overconfidence gets in the way. For most cancers, you have ample time to get a second opinion regarding the type and extent of surgery. Or about whether or not surgery will help. Should you have a mastectomy or a lumpectomy? Should you remove the lung tumor or not? Many of these options are not straightforward, and a decision may require more than one consultation. How many operations like this has the surgeon done recently? What follow-up is required. Will you need to travel far from home? It is very important to be able to use a confident surgeon who is open to having you explore all your options and receive a second opinion. This is not a monogamous relationship. It is important to realize that levels of aggressiveness among surgeons differ greatly. Being aware of their philosophy and experience can prevent misunderstandings and disappointment.

As discussed, few cancers are treated with surgery alone. Most need surgery, chemotherapy, and possibly radiation therapy. You will get a more comprehensive picture of the plan if you are able to meet with all of these specialists before an operation. While such a consultation is not required, you will have fewer surprises and your expectations won't be dashed. Frequently, at larger centers, you may have your case presented at a tumor board, where many specialists are present. Involvement of doctors at these conferences is very helpful to develop a comprehensive plan, but, as noted earlier, **a tumor board does not replace face-to-face consultations**. For example, if you have a throat cancer, you should see the medical and radiation oncologists as well *before* you commit to an operation. Through these consultations, you will get a more thorough understanding about your cancer. Patients are usually very disappointed to learn that there may have been ways to preserve their larynx or voice-box after the operation. At a tumor conference, where all of the appropriate specialists have not personally examined you, bias may be introduced, and plans may be incompletely thought out. An example of such bias is when the majority of physicians who offer an opinion in the case are from only one specialty. Physicians frustrated with the tumor board discussion may unfortunately find it easier to avoid the meeting than to offer honest opinions.

Some operations are done infrequently at local hospitals. A resection of an esophageal tumor is an example. Physicians are somewhat familiar with how to do these surgeries as they are performed in emergencies. You may want to ask if your surgeon would be more comfortable if your esophageal resection is done at a larger center. On the other hand, though, not all surgeries at larger centers are without flaws either. These doctors are sent challenging cases with frequent complications. When a higher complication rate is expected, it is difficult to interpret results. How these larger center surgeons report them can affect how impressive their patients' survival rates appear.

Surgeons, in general, will not be the only physicians doing long-term follow-up for you, the cancer patient. Your medical oncologist and primary care physicians need to be involved. These other doctors will help by screening for other new cancers, watching for long-term complications of treatments, and by monitoring for routine primary care issues. Surgeons are highly focused on the area in which they operate. For example, a urologist will assume that your family doctor will be monitoring you for colon cancer.

Lately surgeons have been offering themselves as experts in certain areas without necessarily having any more training than other surgeons in that field. Often, these are caused by lifestyle choices made by the surgeon. By only doing breast surgery, doctors choose to limit their exposure to other patients with more challenging cases. A general surgeon, however, will not only be able to do your breast surgery, but also will be able to help you with other needs at a later time. These may include bowel complications, need for skin grafts, gall bladder, vascular work, endoscopy, and placing intravenous access catheters. Your local general surgeon is a *key person* with whom you need to have a good working relationship.

It is important to learn the importance of asking if organ preservation is possible, recommended, and worth the price in residual effects. Many new advances in combined modality treatment of cancers allow for more limited surgery and preservation of important organs, such as the larynx, lung, breasts, rectum, and anus. A thorough surgeon will review all of these possibilities with you. However, you should also review them with both your medical and radiation oncologist—before surgery.

The timing of an operation is important. When you come into the doctor's office with cancer, many changes have occurred in your body. You could be malnourished. Your blood may have been altered, and you might be at a much higher risk of getting a blood clot. You could be low on iron and other essential nutrients. Many patients benefit from waiting several months to have surgery. During this time, in addition to addressing the above problems, chemotherapy or radiation treatments are used to treat the tumor. This can often reduce complications, such as blood clots and infections, as well as improve wound healing.

Newer minimally invasive surgical methods that allow for more rapid recovery are expanding across the country. Laparoscopic surgeries are very popular for many reasons. These minimally invasive procedures are done using a tiny telescope and other instruments introduced through small incisions. The recovery time is faster. The scar is smaller. You are back to work quicker. Some problems with this surgery, however, are the limited exams permitted during the surgery. When the surgeon is only able to make a small incision, the field of view through the microscope is compromised. Another problem is the relative novelty of the procedure. It takes a good surgeon time to learn this newer technique.

Craig: Incomplete Staging, Limited Options

Craig was a 60-year-old salesperson who showed up with symptoms of prostate cancer. The PSA (blood) test and the biopsy were consistent with the early stage of the cancer. The radiologist who interpreted the film reported that the cancer might be incurable. The patient, who expected to be offered surgery for an early stage cancer, was shocked when he was told he was incurable. He hadn't lost weight and didn't feel sick. His repeated discussions with the surgeon weren't fruitful, because the surgeon insisted that the bone scan showed metastasis. Metastasis is when a patient's cancer has spread.

When a radiologist suspects cancer on a scan, that concern needs to be confirmed by the clinician—either the surgeon or the oncologist. What occurred in this case happens frequently. No one communicates beyond tests. The physician never picks up the phone.

In Craig's case, the radiologist mentioned spread of the cancer in an effort to include all possible reasons, not as a definitive diagnosis. The radiologist is saying, "This might be cancer."

The surgeon is saying, "I'm going to assume it is." In Craig's case, that was not true. He came to me from a distant city for a second opinion. I agreed that his entire picture was inconsistent with advanced cancer. I then discussed his case with another highly experienced radiologist, who had been made aware of the clinical history. The radiologist reviewed the films and confirmed with a second bone scan that Craig was *not* terminal. What the first radiologist had suggested could be cancer was merely an area of his clothing that had been contaminated with radioactive urine. Craig is relieved and once again pursuing the hope of cure by surgery.

His story illustrates the importance of making sure that your physicians talk to each other, either on the phone or in person, instead of relying only on records. What's in the written record has been vetted through the liability filter. What is expressed verbally might be more honest. It can save your life.

Of course it would be ideal if all of your physicians talked to each other when there is a concern. One obstacle to such conversations is the lack of reimbursement by insurance. Others, such as your lawyer, rarely hesitate to make phone calls for you because they know that payment is expected. In this environment, you need to rely on that good relationship being developed with your oncologist.

RADIATION THERAPY

Radiation treatments take many weeks and require daily trips to a facility. For this reason, most are done as close to home as is possible. For many, it is impractical to consider staying a long distance away for this extended time. While some treatments may take as little as three or four weeks, a total duration of six or seven weeks is not unusual. The normal tissue in your body tolerates radiation therapy best when radiation is given in smaller, divided doses. When given in this manner, your normal tissue can repair itself faster than the cancer can. Newer methods have also been developed, such as gamma knife, cyber knife, or seed implants. that can be done in a single day. Your oncologist can help you know if any of these special types of radiation are appropriate for you.

Radiation is an invisible beam of energy that is used to intensively treat cancer in a specific targeted site of the body. No needles or IVs are involved. You should not expect to lose your hair unless the radiation is being used to treat your brain. The side effects depend on which area of the body is being treated. The goal is to eradicate the cancer in the local region nearby to where your cancer developed. A good example is when radiation is used to treat breast cancer patients. A person might decide to keep a breast. The patient will have a higher than normal risk of the cancer returning in the affected breast if radiation treatments are not used. This will kill the "odd" cancer cells still lurking in the nearby area and treat the area the breast cancer is most likely to return to at a later time.

Patients are frequently confused about whether they will be offered chemotherapy or radiation. You might be treated with both. Radiation therapy is similar to surgery because it only treats the very limited area that is being targeted. It is a local treatment. Chemotherapy, however, is a systemic treatment. Systemic treatments, like chemotherapy or hormone drugs, are treatments that travel throughout the body and are able to kill cancer cells anywhere. It is used to treat your cancer in any of the organs of your body. In our breast cancer example, chemotherapy treatments are used as a means to kill off microscopic deposits of breast cancer in distant organs. Chemotherapy can kill off breast cancer deposits elsewhere in your spine, lung, liver, or brain. On rare occasion, chemotherapy is targeted locally. One example is when chemotherapy can be given directly into the abdominal cavity to treat ovarian cancer. Another is when chemotherapy is administered by a neurosurgeon in wafers near brain tumors. Most uses of chemotherapy, however, are for treatment throughout the entire body.

Radiation and chemotherapy complement each other and can help eradicate the local area of cancer. But the radiation treatments given to your rectum, for example, will not be able to stop the potential spread of rectal cancer to other areas. In some circumstances, though, radiation can be used as the sole method to treat the local area of your cancer. A good example is in lung cancer. Radiation treatments are frequently used to treat lung cancer that has advanced to spread to regional lymph nodes in the chest. Radiation can also be used to help sterilize the region after the surgeon has removed all or part of a tumor. Complete eradication of local cancers, while impossible with chemotherapy, is possible with radiation. Examples include prostate cancer, laryngeal cancer, or lung cancer.

The same radiation treatments that can be deceptively easy in the beginning can be almost cruel when the treatments are nearly over. This is because the side effects depend on the total dose of radiation received by the area of the body being targeted. If your rectum is targeted, you will experience diarrhea and rectal pain. Radiation treatments to a throat cancer will give you a sore throat and trouble swallowing. Your side effects definitely grow increasingly more severe as treatments progress and as you come nearer to your total prescribed dose of radiation. The most severe effects occur during the last two weeks of treatment and the first week or two after they are completed. You might be lulled into a false sense of reassurance by the relative ease of the initial weeks of treatment. Or, you might be falsely reassured by the ease of a friend's radiation treatment. Unfortunately, even if your neighbor breezed through her breast irradiation well, that doesn't always mean that your throat radiation will be as tolerable.

Radiation may be given simultaneously with chemotherapy treatments. This combination kills a larger percentage of cancer cells. Concurrent treatment improves the chances of success. However, if radiation treatments are given along with chemotherapy, there will also be more side effects. Rectal cancer radiation treatments, for example, are frequently and very successfully given along with chemotherapy. The hope is that when radiation is given in this manner, your chances of avoiding a permanent colostomy are better. (A colostomy is an opening in your abdominal wall where stool drains directly from the colon.) Although the combined treatment may result in a higher risk of diarrhea, rectal irritation and pain, most people see this as an acceptable trade off.

Radiation treatments are key in helping patients to preserve organ function. Protocols to use radiation and chemotherapy together for this purpose are commonly used in lung cancer, rectal cancer, and breast cancer. For instance, if you have an advanced throat or laryngeal cancer, preserving your voice may seem important. You may find the option of treatment with chemotherapy and radiation desirable as compared to the surgical option of permanent removal of your voice box and throat.

Luckily, techniques to better protect your normal cells from the effects of radiation have been developed. These include improved ways to target the diseased cells, as well as drugs to limit radiation effects on normal tissue. IMRT or intensity modulated radiation therapy, has been very effective in making radiation more tolerable through careful three-dimensional computerized focusing of the treatment. In this technique, higher doses of radiation can be given with less damage to surrounding normal tissues. IMRT is useful for head and neck cancers, lung cancer, prostate cancer, and breast cancer. Gamma knife and cyber knife are examples of highly focused radiation treatments given over one or a few days.

Radiation therapy treatments are supervised by the radiation therapy physician. These physicians are critical in guiding their team of therapists and physicists in providing treatment. If you need to be hospitalized, however, your oncologist or primary care physician may become involved. These doctors may be better trained to manage the complex medical problems that develop during this period can.

Many long-term effects of radiation treatments exist. It is critical to be aware of these. Wound healing problems in the immediate area are frequent. Radiation treatments affect the small blood vessels in the area that is treated. This results in difficulty healing wounds created in this area. The effect is life-long. An example is men who have had prostate cancer irradiation. Even years after their radiation treatments are done, they will have a very difficult time with surgery in the same area if, for example, they need the removal of a rectal cancer. Excessive amounts of scar tissue left by radiation make the surgeon's job far more challenging and complications much more likely. Only after careful consideration should anyone have an operation in a site that was previously irradiated. Usually this is only done if it has been previously planned. For example, radiation treatments are given before surgery for advanced lung or esophageal cancers.

Another easily overlooked long-term side effect of radiation is the occasional breast cancer patient who has been treated with radiation therapy to the left breast. Depending on her figure and the radiation technique, she may be at a higher risk for heart disease if the heart was exposed to radiation as well. This information may affect your decision about choosing between saving the breast and undergoing radiation therapy or having a mastectomy. You may also benefit from close follow-up for development of underlying heart disease.

CHEMOTHERAPY

For many, chemotherapy ranks only slightly behind cancer itself as something to dread. Many simply refuse treatment and would rather choose death. Patients truly believe that their quality of life will be better by suffering the effects of advancing cancer instead of receiving chemotherapy. It has been widely known that most common cancers. such as lung cancer, pancreatic cancer, and throat cancer, have been very difficult to treat. For this reason, oncologists have pushed the doses of chemotherapy ever and ever higher to the very limits of human tolerability. Unfortunately, oncologists have not always made the tolerability of chemotherapy treatments a high priority. Trying to get the cancer to respond was their highest priority. Often patients suffered severe side effects, including heart damage, lung damage, near fatal infections, kidney failure, extreme nausea, and vomiting. Those who volunteered for the initial studies were usually willing to suffer almost any side effect for a chance to live. Not everyone is. You may be willing to undergo modest inconveniences and side effects, but not extreme ones. All of us have a different limit as to the level of toxicity we are willing to endure in our attempt to survive.

Rarely do oncologists provide patients with in-depth information about how chemotherapy works. Thus, this section is very important, as it will help you understand how cancer acts and responds to treatment. It will also help you to understand the rationale your oncologist uses to order treatments. However, you will need to understand a certain amount of simple biology first.

Chemotherapy is a systemic treatment. Systemic means that the cancer medicine travels throughout your entire body. In most cases, cancer becomes fatal only when it is itself systemic, not local. Brain tumors and throat cancer are examples that could cause death when they are still locally advanced. But most cancers are widespread at the end. Pancreatic cancer, small cell lung cancer, lymphoma, and melanoma are examples of malignancies in which a majority of people show up with distant spread.

Before 1966, no cancer chemotherapy treatments existed that could cure a metastatic cancer (one that has spread). In a landmark study, oncologists combined four drugs, each which was partially effective but could not by itself cure Hodgkin's lymphoma. When combined, however, a high percentage of patients were cured. The drugs were chosen because they had nonoverlapping toxicities. This means that the first drug caused side effects of low blood counts, while another drug might have lung side effects, and a third might have kidney toxicity as its primary side effect. In this way, each drug could then be given at its highest dose. Many other similar combinations of drugs have been developed for a wide variety of cancers. Likewise, only a rare handful of cancers are currently curable with only one chemotherapy drug. One rarely, if ever, kills 100 percent of rapidly dividing cancer cells. For this reason, combinations of chemotherapy drugs are the cornerstone of treatment.

You, like many others, may have thought that chemotherapy is the name of one especially toxic drug. Many patients wrongly believe that a single drug named *chemotherapy* is prescribed by the hour; the sicker you are, the more hours of intravenous treatment you need. Chemotherapy is not one drug, however, but a family of many different anticancer medications. Just like penicillin, tetracycline, and sulfa are all types of antibiotics, many drugs fall into the designation of chemotherapy. If you have metastatic breast cancer, your treatment might include docetaxel, cyclophosphamide, or doxorubicin. If you have bladder cancer, other agents might be used. Non-Hodgkin's lymphoma is treated with cyclophosphamide, adriamycin, vincristine, and prednisone.

These drugs all have their own side effect profiles. Doxorubicin causes hair loss, low blood counts, and mouth sores. Gemzar (gemcitabine) doesn't cause substantial hair loss, but does give some patients low blood counts. Hair loss, nausea, and vomiting are the most common side effects that you may have heard people fear. In the last 10 to 15 years, new drugs have been developed that limit many side effects of chemotherapy and radiation. Hair loss actually occurs with only a few chemotherapy drugs, but it is hard to prevent. Nausea and vomiting, which are common to many chemotherapy agents, are largely preventable with newer nausea drugs, such as ondansetron, Kytril (granisetron), Anzemet (dolasetron) and others, such as Aloxi and Emend. At times, you may need to specifically ask if you are receiving the best nausea medications. Insurance companies will often offer to pay for only modestly effective nausea drugs. Then, if you become sick with initial treatments, they will pay for better ones. Very good medications are available to help control your low blood counts, pain, and nausea and vomiting. Drugs such as Aranesp (darbepoetin), Procrit (epoetin), Neupogen (filgrastim), Neulasta (pegfilgrastim), and Leukine (sargramostim) are approved to help the white and red blood cells recover quicker in certain cancer treatment situations. The billions of dollars of research that have gone into chemotherapy and the years of experience in treating cancer are finally paying off in more tolerable treatments.

FINDING THE CORRECT DOSE

Clinical trials use very precise treatment regimens with specified timetables and doses of medicine. Studies need to be done in this manner to best test scientific theories. But off study, you enjoy far more schedule and dosing flexibility. Most chemotherapy studies have built in dose reductions if you have excessive side effects. Off study you may ask your oncologist to use the opposite technique to find the best dosage. Instead of reducing the dose of chemotherapy for undue side effects, ask if you can try starting your treatments with a more modest dose. You can then raise the dosage as you gain confidence and learn how much you can tolerate. Good theoretical reasons exist to explain why it makes sense to start with the highest amount possible and reduce it for those who can't tolerate it. But, if you are so afraid of being treated that you might refuse treatment, starting with a lower amount makes sense. This way you can be reassured about how tolerable the treatments will be. As you gain confidence and learn about managing side effects, your dose will be increased.

Your oncologist may object to dosing your drugs at minimums because, strictly speaking, they haven't been tested this way. However, the method can be useful in those who are elderly, apprehensive, or have many other complicating medical problems. Clinical trials test patients with only a few other medical problems and those with good health. Many groups of patients, however, have been incompletely tested who still need to be treated further. These include the elderly, minorities, and people with more than one cancer, anxious patients, and rural populations. Such groups have real issues and concerns that require continued study. Often, good clinical judgment on the part of the oncologist can help here.

ADJUVANT CHEMOTHERAPY

Whether or not you consider taking adjuvant chemotherapy (or chemotherapy given in addition to surgery) can be a challenging decision for both your oncologist and you. Adjuvant chemotherapy is similar to an insurance policy. This means that doctors expect to improve the chances that the surgery may have already cured you. This is done by killing off any microscopic deposits of cancer cells. For example, if you have a stage II colon cancer, chemotherapy can be of limited benefit. Patients with stage II colon cancer have a much smaller chance of any microscopic deposits of cancer cells remaining and spreading to become metastatic cancer. If you have a stage III colon cancer, however, the benefit from chemotherapy is clearer because your likelihood of having cancer cells remaining is higher. Both of these are adjuvant uses. Discussions with your oncologist will help you decide if you want to consider this insurance policy of a period of chemotherapy. Similar adjuvant uses of chemotherapy (designed to help ensure that surgery has removed all the cancer) are commonly offered to cancer patients who have breast, lung, or colon cancers. The duration of these treatments has been determined by careful clinical trials. In certain circumstances, the adjuvant chemotherapy is given before the surgery. Your oncologist may have more complicated discussions with you about the timing, benefit, and duration of your adjuvant chemotherapy based on your individual situation. Clinical trials are looking into other important uses for adjuvant chemotherapy, such as in men with prostate cancer.

Bill: Needed More Options

Bill, a 75-year-old farmer, initially presented with early stage colon cancer (several years earlier.) Bill wasn't convinced about the usefulness of chemotherapy treatments to prevent his colon cancer from spreading (these treatments usually last about six months). As he was feeling well at the time, Bill chose not to be treated with chemotherapy. Within two years, however, his cancer had spread to his lungs and liver. Needing relief from pain near his liver, Bill decided to receive treatment. He was treated with chemotherapy which relieved his pain. He survived another three years before entering hospice care for four months. If he had been offered and accepted six months of adjuvant chemotherapy treatments immediately after his surgery, his cancer might never have spread. A short course of treatment at that time could have been far easier to tolerate, been more effective, and might have prevented the ultimate spread of his cancer.

METASTATIC CANCER

Often chemotherapy is used to treat the symptoms of widespread cancer. If you have metastatic prostate cancer, you might be offered a single drug called taxotere. Sometimes drug combinations are used to relieve cancer-related symptoms. For metastatic lung cancer, a combination of two drugs, alimta and cisplatin, may be offered. I am often asked by patients with metastatic cancer, "*How many months will I be on treatment?*" A little math is needed to understand the answer. Let's discuss.

Chemotherapy Math Simplified

As you begin treatment with symptoms of metastatic cancer, the total body burden of cancer cells is high, usually very high. When treatment is started, tens of billions of cancer cells might be causing symptoms. At a time when a cancer patient is near death, he may have greater than 100 billion cancer cells. Testicular cancer and lymphoma are examples of types of cancer that are especially sensitive to chemotherapy. Luckily, a particularly high number, perhaps greater than 99 percent of these types of cancer cells, are killed with each chemotherapy cycle. Unfortunately, for most other cancers, chemotherapy can, at best, only kill a much smaller number of the cancer cells inside you. When your burden of cancer cells reaches somewhere less than 1 billion cells, your symptoms of cough, pain, or shortness of breath will likely go away. For most cancers, it is challenging for even the best X-ray or lab test to detect when someone has a small number of cancer cells.

But remember, even as you are being treated with chemotherapy, the cancer will try to grow. Many chemotherapy drugs are most effective and at their highest concentration for several days after treatment is received — only. The drug may be out of the system and can't be detected in the blood stream, but its effects on the body and system remain. Because many chemotherapy drugs affect your blood counts, they also can't be given too often. At this time, the cancer may resume growing as you and your body and blood counts recover.

Thus, each cycle of treatment may result in only a small decrease in the total number of cancer cell inside you. Or, your condition may become a stalemate with the rate of cancer cells dying being equal to the growth rate of the cancer. This explains why it may take many cycles of treatment to gain control over your cancer. It also explains why early detection is so important.

How Long?

You need to be the one to decide if you are being helped by chemotherapy. Give it some time, though. The cancer probably has been growing for five or ten years, and it won't change overnight. One useful analogy is that turning around the growth of an advanced lung cancer is similar to turning around a large ocean liner—it doesn't turn as fast as your lawn mower does. Is your pain getting better? Is your breathing better? Are you taking fewer pain pills? Many times people don't remember how bad they felt. Gradual changes should be expected, not dramatic ones. If symptoms don't worsen in the first several months that means you're making progress if you have an aggressive cancer. If your metastatic cancer has a complete response to your chemotherapy treatments (meaning that all evidence of your cancer has left), stopping them and observing is a reasonable approach. But it is very important to remember one important point. Retreating cancer is not nearly as easy as treating it the first time. Treating someone who has previously received chemotherapy is far more challenging. This is because your cancer develops drug resistance. The initial cancer that presented is usually populated with relatively sensitive cells. The cancer that recurs after your treatment has been stopped for a while is usually heavily populated with resistant cancer cells.

Who Picks the Drugs?

For each type of cancer, several equivalent combinations of drugs may exist. The deciding factor may not always be the side effects or your specific health situation. Financial concerns may also play a role. Newer chemotherapy drugs are very expensive. They are big business. Clinics, hospital systems, insurers, and large cancer centers all have complex financial arrangements that affect the profit margin for medications. Any physician or clinic is paid similarly for each specific drug. However, each provider pays a different rate to acquire the drugs. Although recent changes have helped to limit this problem, incentives could encourage physicians to use one drug over another. In this way, one product can gain the largest market share. You may be completely unaware of such arrangements. Unless you ask. Ask your oncologist. Does the system encourage the use of one drug over another? Is this really the best drug for you as an individual or is it the one being pushed by *the system* this quarter? Expect a very complicated answer. But if your type of cancer has several options of treatment that are equally acceptable, the hospital or clinic should not be using mainly one product. If they are using a predominance of one drug, that may be a sign that financial concerns are interfering with medical decisions. This also applies to supportive care drugs for nausea, vomiting, antibiotics etc.

TREATMENT GUIDELINES

Experts have developed treatment guidelines to help standardize current cancer care. Using the best data and research, these guidelines are available for many common cancers and circumstances. Some diseases or situations have not been studied sufficiently to give a doctor the information needed to advise a patient. In these circumstances, judgment and experience are important guides. If an oncologist has relatively limited experience for whatever reason or if she is accustomed to only using treatment guidelines, she may be challenged to make recommendations. She may also suggest getting second and even third opinions. Being open to getting these is great, but often you need someone to *decide* because you need to start something *now*.

There is no substitute for experience. Lots of experience. In many large centers, where there are highly trained, very specialized, and respected physicians, only a few are actually in the clinic seeing patients. Oddly, for many physicians gaining such experience is not always a priority. The work put into a relationship with an oncologist can serve a patient well here. Treatment recommendations are educated guesses. Guidelines are not perfect. Many new developments have come about because some brave proactive oncologist has not limited his treatments to only approved guidelines and has tried something, anything, in a desperate situation. Clinical trials may not fit every situation. Patients don't have the time or money to drive to where the trials are. They can't always wait to be approved for a study.

EMPOWER YOURSELF

You have learned that cancer treatments may not be as difficult as you once thought. A serious discussion often involves looking into surgery, radiation, and chemotherapy.

The latest surgery techniques offer the hope of organ preservation and better reconstruction methods. Understanding the surgeon's comments after the operation is also crucial.

Modern radiation machines are better able to treat cancer by improved dosing to only the cancer and not normal surrounding tissues. Even so, radiation treatments have challenges, such as delayed wound healing and fatigue.

Chemotherapy is not one drug but many, each with its own side effects. Newer administrative methods such as weekly treatments may be more tolerable.

WHAT'S NEXT

Major pharmaceutical companies have been exposed for their profit motives and expensive drugs. But they also can help you during your treatment in many ways. Learn how.

Chapter 9

The Pharmaceutical Industry
Friend or Foe?

Anyone diagnosed with cancer needs to take a close look at the multi-billion dollar pharmaceutical industry and the part it plays in the cancer system. You have probably heard more negatives than positives about the role of drug companies in cancer treatment. It is said that they're heartless, solely profit driven, and spend a great deal of money on marketing and courting the favor of physicians. Anyone who's seen or heard about the Michael Moore film, *SiCKO*, knows that the cancer pharmaceutical industry is big business.

INVESTOR AND CANCER PATIENT

It is true that the efforts of drug companies are directed at getting the best return for their investors. Why not? This is their stated purpose. And usually the investors are all of us. Millions of everyday people own a small part of the drug companies through retirement accounts. Together we demand that they strive to get us the best possible return on our money. If they don't, then we sell their stock and buy some other. True, they're not charitable organizations.

There are a plethora of reasons why they need to charge as much as they do for their drugs. Expensive basic science research, costly clinical trials, and volumes of regulatory documents needed for drug approval are some of the reasons for the expense of the drugs. Some agents fall into a special category, where much of the expense is related to specific liability worries. Others associated with serious risks may have a substantial amount of legal costs built into the price. Newer drugs may need months of complicated molecular design and development in the lab before being tested in animals. Some of these compounds that look favorable in the lab frequently are found ineffective when tested in animals or humans. This all adds quite a bit to expenses. Compounds that are tested favorably in animals or humans may not be useful because of problems with their ability to remain stable on the shelf and be effectively stored. Finally, a compound that has been studied may have trouble with its side effect profile.

As businesses with stockholders to report to, pharmaceutical houses have to take on projects that give them a reasonable return. They take tremendous risks, often investing hundreds of millions of dollars in research and development on a single drug before it becomes apparent that it's really going to work. According to the *New York Times*, for example, Genentech claims to have spent $2.25 billion, along with its partner Roche, on developing its drug Avastin. Also according to the November 10, 2007 issue of *Business Week*, the pharmaceutical industry launched 19 new drugs in 2007, with $59 billion spent on research and development! Clearly these are large sums to invest.

WAYS PHARMACEUTICAL COMPANIES CAN HELP YOU

After fifteen years of dealing closely with these companies, I've realized that on a day-to-day basis, they can be helpful to my patients. Although I'm well aware that the drug representatives are there to market to me, I try to refocus the relationship on the many ways their enormous resources can directly benefit my patients. You should know that the pharmaceutical industry is highly regulated and that any clinical trials, support programs, or marketing efforts are initiated only with the approval and oversight of the FDA.

For example, many companies have resources available to grant to local not-for-profit cancer support groups to assist with their educational programs. These programs often provide general information regarding the particular cancer and are not specific marketing efforts related to the drug being sold. The representative's efforts can also be redirected by asking the company for information regarding its indigent programs that provide free drugs to poor patients. Other areas in which they may be able to help are providing background information for staff regarding a particular type of cancer being treated.

Another resource they can bring to the office environment is to provide research assistance to the physician. This may be as simple as asking the company to provide a review of all of the research that has been done by others.

Not only are pharmaceutical companies leaders in developing new cancer drugs, but they're helpful in many indirect ways. About half of all the money spent on cancer research is provided by drug companies. These companies have the potential to provide help for a great number of people. Every time I am visited by a representative, I try to get some help for my patients. Your doctor may find you benefit in the same ways I do mine. Here is an example.

Amos: No Insurance and in Remission

Amos was a 60-year-old restaurant owner whose beliefs kept him from owning insurance. Money wasn't the issue; he just didn't believe in it. Amos was a member of a religious community that had always provided for the heath care of its members. Insurance was felt to be unnecessary and might be seen as a lack of faith. If necessary, the larger group of many affiliated churches would help pay for expenses.

Still, when he developed an aggressive and usually fatal metastatic cancer, he was overwhelmed by the potential bills. He initially refused the treatment as he didn't want to bankrupt his family and church, both of which had offered to help him pay for the care.

A solution was found when he was started on an oral drug used to treat melanoma. A foundation, which was set up to help those unable to afford the drug, allowed him access to the drug for free based on his limited income. During the time he was provided the drug, other arrangements were made to provide long-term insurance.

EDUCATION

PHYSICIAN EDUCATION

As each new chemotherapy drug arrives on the market, drug companies try to arrange help for an oncologist to learn how to safely use them.

At times, companies will send trained experts directly to the local oncologist's office to review interactions with other drugs, educate pharmacy and nursing staff, and bring big center experience to a local oncologist office. Having an experienced person on site is reassuring to the patient, family, staff, and physician. An oncologist may also be more confident about using a new drug as he learns from the experience of other physicians who have studied the drug,

Sponsor Physician Education Projects

Companies are usually willing to organize physician educational efforts aimed at either the treating oncologist or the primary physician. These symposia are available and usually provide timely information. Physician continuing educational credits are provided, thereby increasing the likelihood of participation among doctors. By enhancing community awareness about the treatment of specific diseases, these efforts can help you. I've even had educational talks given that are initiated for the benefit of one individual patient. The chance for successful treatment depends on the medical community developing local oncologists with up-to-date knowledge.

Obtain Funding for Support Groups, Patient Education Efforts, and Community Projects

While strict new federal rules exclude pharmaceutical companies from directing any revenue intended to help patient support groups through physician's offices, monies still exist for many similar benevolent purposes. Most large pharmaceutical companies have voluntarily entered into compliance with industry-sponsored guidelines that limit grants, travel expenses, and gifts to physicians. These well-intentioned guidelines serve the public successfully. Companies are also still willing and able to provide support directly to the cancer patient community. Instead of pens and pads to the physicians, they provide scarves and hand warmers to support groups to give to patients receiving chemotherapy. The key is that the effort needs to help the patients and their non-profit community support groups.

When not-for-profit groups request funding directly for patient education, it is more likely to be approved. Examples of some programs include education about screening for breast cancer, help for survivors dealing with money crises, or treatments to help patients tolerate therapies better. Requests may need to be made yearly or specifically for certain projects. Gloves to help patients whose hands are cold and numb, requests for wigs or scarves, money to help a bone marrow donor drive, or money to help fund a support groups are examples of specific helpful projects. Pharmaceutical companies may also be more likely to direct funds to projects that have a connection to their drugs. A company with a breast cancer drug may thus be most interested in a support group effort to increase the number of women screened by mammograms.

Obtain Books, Educational Videos, and Patient Resources

Many approved educational books, videos, audiotapes, and other resources may be provided to help patients, family members, and others understand various cancers. These products may be focused directly at a specific cancer connected to the company's product. I have had patients provided directly with gloves, blankets, thermometers, and other products useful for everyday life. Companies are permitted to supply similar products that directly help patients.

Find Researchers and Physician Experts

Drug companies keep listings of physicians with whom they have worked with and who are experienced in the use of a certain drug. Often these physicians are some of the early users, who have the most experience using the new agent. Their experience is important and may help to reassure an oncologist on how to safely administer the drug and for which patients it would be most appropriate. It's important to seek out a second opinion consultation with one of these experienced more specialized physicians.

Connect to Physicians Distant From You

Various pharmaceutical company representatives have helped my patients by connecting me with established and reputable doctors in other states. Patients who have asked for my help finding physicians in other regions know that this is one of the ways to find established oncologists. With their inside track on a physician's tenure, reputation, and status in the oncology community, this method has become a continued source of good physician referrals to my patients in distant locales. Here's how it works. A local drug company representative contacts his partner in a distant state. The local rep's extensive knowledge of the available physicians is then used to find the most trusted oncologist in the region to which a patient will be moving or visiting. While it's important to recognize that there may be a bias in their opinion toward a particular type of physician, many of my patients who spend the winter in warmer climates have been happy with the oncologists they have found this way.

INFORMATION SHARING

As discussed, the pharmaceutical representative is an important source of information sharing among offices. He may bring data about local educational opportunities to the oncologist and his staff. Disease-related lectures for the hospital and clinic staff, held locally, can benefit someone directly and indirectly. Pharmaceutical companies are also aware of where drugs are in the developmental process and in what manner they may be made available. Ask your oncologist for information from the company regarding the status of any drugs you might need. Pharmaceutical reps are also good sources of information regarding insurer payment for a particular new treatment.

Some breakthrough biological drugs which are FDA approved for use in several common types of advanced or metastatic cancers patients have also been found to be useful in other patients, including some lung cancer patients. These drugs are given in the vein like standard chemotherapy, but kill the cancer in a much different manner than does standard chemotherapy. They work by effecting small areas called receptors on the surface of cancer cells. The fact that several different cancers will respond to one biologic drug makes sense because often two different cancers share similar biologic features. (I know I'm being vague and have not given you the names of these drugs, but your oncologist will know to which drugs I'm referring. Stricter federal rules make it complicated to mention the use of a drugs for a cancer treatment that the FDA has not yet approved.) While extensive research has been done and their use is considered by many oncologists and numerous major groups, not all Medicare regional carriers agree. These regional carriers have the discretion to decide locally whether to pay for the new use of this biologic drug. At the time of this writing, patients in approximately half the country are permitted to have these drugs paid for by Medicare.

This is because before a drug receives a specific FDA indication, there may be inconsistencies throughout the country. As a result, the drug may be paid for in one region, but not another. In the complex dance between the patient and an insurance company or Medicare—a dance that is now unfortunately part of the oncologist's and patient's world—this information is essential. If patients in another state are able to receive a certain treatment, why are you not able to do the same? This information will help a doctor best advocate for the patient. An assertive proactive oncology office will develop a professional relationship with its local Medicare carrier and strongly advocate for you to get access to the drugs you deserve.

Information may also flow the other way. A drug rep can also take back to the industry important observations that community physicians have made when using a new drug. Even after one is approved, many side effects can occur. Some new biological drugs, such as Erbitux (cetuximab) that is used for colon cancer, have a curious tendency to be associated with drug reactions during its infusion, but only in certain areas of the country. Information from many hospitals and physicians' offices was used to develop a method to premedicate patients to avoid this reaction. Your local oncologist brings a tremendous wealth of experience, knowledge, and intuition to the discussion. At times, this results in the development of a technique to more safely administer the drug.

By relaying information similar to this to the company, we were able to share this new technique with other physicians' offices. Often, it is only after a drug is used for several years that the ideal dose and schedule is truly understood. Many examples can be given in which the FDA-approved dose and schedule are not the ones most oncologists feel comfortable using. While drug company literature will always suggest the FDA-approved dose, other alternative schedules have been studied and are available through the company.

ONCOLOGY SOCIETIES

The costs of organizing many local and national oncology associations and their foundations, such as the American Society of Clinical Oncology (ASCO) are substantially funded by pharmaceutical companies, such as Genentech, Glaxo, and Novartis and Sanofi-Aventis. Member dues and other sources of funding contribute only a modest amount of the money needed to run these organizations, which have research, educational, and advocacy roles. The resources made available by the drug companies help further these goals. Part of your oncologist's training may have involved grants to sponsor cancer research as a result of a drug company's financial support.

COMPASSIONATE AVAILABILITY OF CHEMOTHERAPY

Most patients are amazed that the cost of new cancer drugs can be several thousand dollars a month regardless of whether the drug is given intravenously or orally. All chemotherapy drugs given in the vein are administered in the office in the presence of a physician. Never are they administered in the home setting. A charge to cover the intravenous administration in the office is routinely added. Even though some cancer medicines can be administered orally, this hasn't decreased the cost. You are paying largely for the safety and effectiveness of the drug regardless of how it is given. Rarely are generics available. When these drugs are used indefinitely and alongside a host of many other necessary drugs, the costs escalate further. Even with only a 10 percent or 20 percent copay, the price can be prohibitive. But it's wrong to assume that a patient won't have access to expensive drugs if there is no insurance. Don't give up before you ask for assistance. Your oncology office should be able to advocate for you and get free drugs through the company that manufactures them. But note that many physician groups will avoid taking on the added bureaucratic expense and headache involved in going through this process.

You may be surprised to learn that most companies have programs that make many drugs available without charge. Our office employs staff members who work with drug companies, foundations, local support groups, and anyone else to help our patients gain access to needed medication. Usually the people who work in this office feel great about their jobs because they enjoy helping patients. One of our staff even has a superhero poster hanging above her computer. While not all offices will provide this service, it is a sign of a proactive concerned office if it does. For many reasons, including privacy, timeliness, and technical knowledge, this essential role cannot be done by volunteers from support groups. It is part of the unpaid goodwill that the physician's office gives to the community. The pharmaceutical companies, by the way, are very resourceful and almost always make it possible to obtain the needed drug. If you meet their financial criteria, the companies will often provide the drugs indefinitely.

It is a rare patient who is prepared to face a financial strain as large as cancer. Patients often need work done on estate or financial planning to qualify for programs. After the shock of having cancer wears off, they may need to obtain the advice of social workers, accountants, and attorneys. Preparing the extensive paperwork needed to apply for these drug programs almost forces you to go through the estate planning process. It is good to get this process completed.

To benefit from the free drug programs, you and your oncologist must meet special requirements. You apply to the programs through your oncologist's office. Although there are fairly liberal income and asset requirements that differ with each drug company, they usually require that the physician administer the drugs for free. Both intravenous and oral drugs are available. Sometimes a benevolent oncology office will offer this service, but not every oncologist's office will be willing to participate by administering the drugs for free. The reason is that the oncologist is not receiving payment to defray overhead and staffing, so that it actually costs money to treat you for free. These programs do, however, take much of the financial strain off of you and your provider when the expensive medications are made available. You may need to be referred to another office if your oncologist won't provide this service.

PAYMENT ADVOCACY

Drug companies will also help advocate to get your treatment paid for when insurance problems arise. Again, this help is given through your oncologist's office. The staff makes the initial contact, and then a representative contacts you. These representatives work for businesses contracted by pharmaceutical companies to provide support services. Some of the larger types of these groups are:

Genentech-Access Solutions
Glaxo-Smith Kline-Commitment to Access
Amgen Safety Net
Lilly-Lilly oncology reimbursement
Bristol-Meyers Squibb/Imclone-Destination Access
Pfizer-Connection to Care
Celgene-Access Solutions

The pharmaceutical industry has established many programs with the specific responsibility of strongly advocating for your interests. When an expensive drug is used for an off-label purpose, you may wish to prepare ahead of time to prevent problems. (Off-label use is when a drug already on the market for colon cancer, for example, is given to a patient with another type of cancer.) The oncologist might believe that new data supports its use. By registering your use with the drug company program, the oncologist's office greatly improves the chance that you will not have to pay personally if there is a problem.

It is important, therefore, to have all of the data justifying the off-label use of a drug. At times, your insurance will fail to pay for such cancer treatments. They aren't always your best advocate in helping you receive the latest therapy. Only when pushed do some pay. The insurance companies will strictly interpret treatment guidelines and indications to their advantage, not yours. By strictly interpreting the official language in the drug's approval guideline, the insurance company may try to restrict your treatment. The insurer's can be very inflexible. To counter this, some programs will find the latest medical research that backs your oncologists suggested use of the drugs. With this information, your treatment is far more likely to be paid for. If you find out that a treatment has not been approved, try asking your oncologist to recruit some help.

PHYSICIAN-INITIATED RESEARCH

University professors study a very limited group of carefully selected patients. Your local oncologist, however, benefits from the experience of caring for a more diverse group of patients in the community. When this larger more diverse experience leads to an important observation, he can approach drug companies to sponsor a research study. Some of these observations may include methods of using various premedications to limit chemotherapy side effects. Other important observations include different drug administration schedules that make drugs more amenable to real-life situations. These ideas may include changing from a once-a-month to a lower once-a-week dose. In a similar way, your local oncologist can take his observations and develop them into useful clinical trials. Only a small number of oncologists will take advantage of this opportunity. The backing of the drug company helps by giving logistical and financial support as well as by providing the drugs. In this way, the experience of your oncologist can lead to important developments.

ENROLL IN A DRUG COMPANY-SPONSORED STUDY

Drug companies need to spend a lot of money developing their drugs for approval. Every patient in every study becomes important. Depending on the drug company sponsor, resources may be available to pay for travel, medical, and other expenses. Once you are accepted for a clinical trial, the company will go to great efforts to keep you from dropping out. One of our patients, for example, was picked up at home and driven to the clinic for a lab test in a storm to comply with the study requirements. Another had number of medical bills paid for by the study sponsor. Drugs that are considered experimental are routinely provided without charge. Sometimes, they will continue to be given free even after FDA approval.

Many years of clinical trials studying thousands of patients are required to receive FDA approval for a new drug. Newer biological drugs, such as Avastin, have cost over 2 billion dollars to develop. The dollars spent on such trials turn into a good investment only if the treatment is successful. Far more support dollars are available for these studies than for government-sponsored studies.

ONCOLOGY DRUG COMPANY CONCERNS

There are several concerns common to oncology pharmaceutical companies. These include the type of cancers they choose to study, an overemphasis on profits, and close ties to university research.

DRUG COMPANY OVEREMPHASIS
ON COMMON CANCERS

Intense market pressures to produce company profits often brings about the availability of new drugs for common cancers, and this immediately helps afflicted patients. Several drug companies may be simultaneously developing new drugs for the more common cancers, such as lung, breast, and colon cancers. Research into the development of new drugs for less common cancers, however, occurs less often. If someone has a less common cancer, such as mesothelioma or a brain tumor, the patient may have to wait longer for new products to be developed or be made available.

Off-label use can provide some opportunities for treatment. For example, biologic drugs approved for use in one type of advanced colon cancer have now found use in some aggressive brain tumors. This type of use is called off label. Companies may choose not to pursue approvals for off-label treatments, as these approvals are becoming more expensive each year. Whether or not to pursue FDA approval for a particular indication is often a business, and not a medical, decision. A drug may be a very effective treatment for an uncommon tumor, yet lack an official indication. Seeking approval may just not be cost effective. Physicians have to be knowledgeable about these drugs before administering them. Off-label use needs to be justified by available clinical research.

Extremely large profits on current drugs help explain why companies have such tremendous interest in taking such risks in developing new cancer drugs.

DRUG COMPANIES ARE PROFIT DRIVEN

Because of the intensive pressure to show quarterly profits, drug companies focus their marketing and development efforts on the short term. The result is an emphasis on marketing already available drugs for the treatment of the more common cancers, as well as the treatment of common side effects. This profit motive also drives the race to intensely market their most expensive new drugs to physicians. Resulting billion dollar sales figures motivate other companies to seek out similar lucrative markets.

Simultaneously, regulators are watching the same sales figures with an eye toward tighter guidelines over the use of such expensive drugs. These restrictions brought about by the intense regulatory oversight then has the effect of limiting the use of otherwise effective drugs.

CLOSE TIES TO UNIVERSITY RESEARCH

The oncologists who carry out chemotherapy research at major universities and cancer centers have complex and intimate ties to pharmaceutical companies. Consulting and advisory relationships are often established that include speaker's fees, research grants, participation on advisory boards, and educational symposium. Much of a university's financial support for labs and salaries is closely tied to these large companies. As a result, concerns exist over conflicts of interest. Despite regulatory scrutiny, this relationship between researchers and drug companies can affect nuances in the studies. Many choices, including how the studies are designed and the choice of drugs, might be affected.

TIES TO CORPORATE ONCOLOGY

The world of corporate oncology offices is affected by the market penetration of various chemotherapy drugs. Small differences in the expense of each chemotherapy drug can affect profits at both the corporate oncology office and the pharmaceutical company. A few top tier physicians, who hold positions of authority in corporate oncology, are able to limit and prioritize treatment decisions for many physicians. To be most efficient, drug companies focus their marketing efforts toward these executive oncologists. While appropriate drugs are given, options are deliberately curtailed. Again, complex consultative and advisory relationships may exist. The spirit of laws meant to limit conflicts of interest may be compromised. Patients who develop a close relationship with their oncologist can hope to have a better opportunity to see all of the options.

DRUG COMPANY REGULATORY ISSUES

Drug companies have major restraints—both regulatory and liability-wise—on their behavior. This means that the information they provide to you is essentially limited to only the FDA-approved package insert, which is the only information approved by the agency for dissemination to the public.

Regulatory agencies are intensely interested in defending their decisions on whether to approve or withdrawal agents, particularly since the public reviews their efforts. The importance of public reaction is far more apparent if a regulatory agency approves a drug that has serious side effects. The public routinely accepts delays in the approval of a new drug to help those who are suffering from a serious cancer. For some reason, the public is more forgiving of such delays than it is of problems with a new drug. Monitoring drugs for undetected side effects is an important regulatory responsibility after a drug is approved and on the market. It is also part of the oncologist's role to monitor and report these effects.

Although these agencies face a challenging and difficult task, rarely do they step out on a limb for the cancer patient. Drug companies tend to be more proactive in moving cancer advances forward and more interested in wanting the patient to receive treatment. They have a more direct stake in rates of survival. Here, the profit motive helps. While others, such as universities or federal agencies, may discover a drug, it takes a major drug firm to develop it, produce it, get it approved, and bring it successfully to market. If you lack access to the drugs you need, the fault could lie more often with the regulatory agencies than with the drug companies.

EMPOWER YOURSELF

Major pharmaceutical companies, such as Bristol Myers Squib, Genentech, Amgen, Roche, Pfizer, Sanofi-Aventis, have enormous resources. Tapping into these resources may assist you on your journey. This help may be in the form of direct support or through the community backing of physicians, research, and oncology societies. Their enormous research budgets help extensive networks of studies, some of which may benefit you.

WHAT'S NEXT

In the next chapter, you'll learn the best ways to give yourself every chance to survive. From the obvious suggestion to quit smoking to the less obvious ones of speaking up, voicing concerns clearly, and not hiding from the process.

Chapter 10

Making Your Own Luck
Tested Ways to Improve Survival Chances

C ancer patients need to be at the top of their games. Paying attention to all those details and being disciplined is a serious challenge when someone feels terrible. But you now know that patients need to be proactive, organized, and ready to fight. They need to seek out, listen to, and follow good advice. They also need to believe that they will live, not that they are doomed. Persistence matters. You need to get back up, even if you sometimes confront failures. No one is perfect. This chapter will explain specific ways in which patients can help themselves. Every detail in this chapter could, in fact, be critical.

Avoid the attitude that one patient showed to me. Lenny had long complained about his lack of energy. When he was asked to undergo testing to determine how to treat his underlying condition, known as sleep apnea, he refused and said, "I've got so many problems now that I can't deal with any more."

Lenny was obviously overwhelmed by all of his medical problems, but facing them is important. Lenny's attitude did nothing to erase the fatigue, body aches, and irritability from sleep deprivation. Only by undergoing the testing would he increase his survival chances. Finally, after agreeing to the testing and receiving the CPAP breathing treatment, he felt much stronger.

Perhaps you have been blessed with excellent health. With little effort you have enjoyed many good years. But life can change. Making your health a priority at this time is obviously critical. Your attitude can't be the one that a patient wore proudly on his t-shirt throughout his treatment: *Whatever*. Treatment means more than simply going to the physician for exams and medication. It means taking charge of your life and helping the oncologist take better care of you. Pay attention to your body. Make notes. Observe honestly. Don't deny. Report changes. How far can the you walk? How much weight have you lost? How much exertion can you really handle? How much pain are you really experiencing? It is not unusual for patients to underreport their own pain. Some symptoms that may appear to be an exacerbation of an existing problem may actually reflect a new problem. For example, a person who has had back pain for years should report any new back pains, as they have a separate cause. This information will help the oncologist tremendously in his evaluation.

THE GRIEF CYCLE

Everyone who is diagnosed with a serious life-threatening condition like cancer can be expected to grieve. People naturally start to grieve for the loss of good health. No one is exempt. It helps if you understand the five stages of grief: denial, anger, bargaining, depression, and acceptance. Knowing where you are in this chain of expected reactions will help you move through to the most functional stage, the fifth one called acceptance. By accepting your condition, you are able to make plans, to adjust, and to avoid behavior that is not constructive. By deciding to read this book, a person with cancer moved past the first stage, which is denial.

It is very heart wrenching to see someone stuck in the denial stage because you are watching someone's cancer progress when it might be treatable. Physicians naturally feel uneasy when they have to sit idly by and watch a treatable cancer progress for this reason. A patient who persists in denying his or her condition should not be surprised if a physician doesn't offer return appointments.

The second stage, anger, is also unhealthy for the patient, as it makes one constantly irritable. This will only serve to alienate physicians, nurses, and friends who are trying to help. Yes, a good physician may recognize your pain and see through it, but not all have the time or willingness to empathize. Remember that you are trying to improve your relationship with all of these people. Being angry at the cancer is expected. Being angry at fate is okay. Being angry at the people trying to help you is counterproductive and a very bad idea. Channel or subvert that energy somewhere else. Paint. Meditate. Pray. Garden. Exercise. But don't get thrown out of the radiology department for yelling at the mammogram technician. If you are one of those people who can naturally divert your frustrations elsewhere, you are lucky. If not, you will need to learn from others. Take a class. Do something. Just don't take it out on your caregivers.

Not all oncologists are able to recognize that a patient is only venting while going through the stages of grieving. Oncologists are human also. They all bring an assortment of their own issues to the relationship. While they have been trained and should recognize the anger that naturally occurs with the grief process, some physicians may react with their own anger. Others may see the situation as simply a matter of efficiency. Your care takes a lot more time if you are stuck in the anger phase of grieving over the loss of your own health,

Bargaining is the next step in the grief process. It is easy to remain stuck here for many years. During this phase, people will often set themselves up to be amateur physicians. Comments like these are a tip-off: "I don't think that I need this chemotherapy drug, just a little time." Or "I won't come back for a lab or X-ray in three months, maybe in a year. Can I only do a CAT scan and not a PET scan? Do I have to do six months of treatment? Will four months do?"

To be sure there are many legitimate reasons for people opting against certain therapies. These include not being able to tolerate or afford them, or simply deciding against certain treatments. But in the bargaining phase of grief, every single recommendation is a protracted negotiation. It is reminiscent of haggling at a flea market. Some oncologists tire of this behavior and tend to offer the least aggressive and most conservative treatments. At other times, they refuse to offer any treatment as the patient has not completely engaged in their recommendations. Because the success of cancer treatments is based on following complex treatment algorithms, they may also simply opt out of treating a patient altogether. Your oncologist can most accurately quote to you the chances of curing your Hodgkin's lymphoma if your treatment closely follows the protocol that was studied. If you constantly delay, reduce doses, and drop drugs, it is hard to know what your chance of a cure are. You oncologists is most confident that he is helping you when he can closely follow a detailed protocol that was extensively studied.

The fourth stage of grief, depression, is the most challenging to get through. It is just about impossible to treat a severely or chronically depressed person. This is regardless of whether it is a reaction to being diagnosed with cancer. Recognizing the depression and the need for psychological treatment is an enormous step. Frequently, others will be better able to recognize a patient's depression. Lack of energy, lack of motivation, trouble concentrating, and trouble sleeping are some of the common signs. If a person is very depressed, sometimes the only strategy is to take several weeks time to treat just the emotions. When patients are depressed, they don't see any reason to treat their diseases. Unfortunately, depressed patients will actually unexpectedly welcome the death that comes with cancer almost as a friend. It allows them a passive and socially acceptable way to pass away. The cancer can do what they may not have been able to do themselves but may have considered, which is to cause their own death. This is different than acceptance. When a depressed patient refuses therapy that has a high chance of success, depression, not cancer, is the most immediate cause of death. For example, untreated cancers, such as lymphoma, small cell lung cancer and metastatic breast cancer, all have a high chance of initial success with limited side effects. However, it is not unusual for a depressed patient with these cancers to refuse to walk up to the plate and try even one therapy.

At times it appears that depressed patients have the following attitude, "I don't have to take any action at all. My being completely passive will result in my death." Many will completely refuse any treatment. Or, they may prematurely seek to enter a hospice. They see no hope. No light at the end of the tunnel. Only potential side effects and more of an unpleasant current situation are expected. If life without cancer was depressing and almost unbearable, then life with cancer is unthinkable for them.

Depression is a disorder of energy. Patients don't have the emotional energy to fight. When depressed, patients assume that they will get all of the side effects and that the treatment won't work. The glass is always half empty. With a positive attitude, people find ways to deal with side effects as they come up. Recognizing and admitting the depression is the first step. It is critical to get effective treatment. Numerous effective strategies exist, including medication and counseling. You need only ask for help, but many patients ask for help in ways that not all doctors recognize. While patients may be reluctant to tell their oncologist *I am depressed*, they will frequently put it in their own terms and say, *I have no energy*. In addition, it is hard for a patient mired in depression or anger to have the ability to bond with his or her oncologist.

True acceptance occurs when patients begin to participate in plans to address their cancer. Consultations happen, questions get asked, and decisions get made. This is not easy, but it allows a deep and sincere bond to develop with the oncologist.

QUIT SMOKING

Quit smoking. Completely. It is a simple as that. Quitting smoking (or any tobacco use) is the simplest way to improve one's chances of preventing or treating cancer. The bad effects of smoking that contribute to your chances of getting cancer may continue for ten to twenty years after you quit. In addition, smoking has a negative effect on cancer treatment. My observations over many years suggest that smokers do not respond as effectively to chemotherapy or radiation therapy. One reason might be that smoking may affect your body's metabolism of cancer drugs. Another reason is that smokers have a much higher rate of atherosclerosis and other diseases that can limit wound healing. The risks of surgical complications are greater as well. Wounds don't heal because they aren't getting enough blood supply. Also, just having cancer greatly increases the chances of a serious blood clot or stroke. Since smoking also typically increases blood clots in the legs and lungs, the combination greatly increases chances of stroke and heart attacks. Chewing tobacco is similarly bad for your health and is not regarded as any safer than smoking. While chewing tobacco has its greatest effect on the throat, the chemicals in the tobacco are absorbed into the bloodstream and can affect the entire body.

The physiological effects of smoking are extensive. Chemotherapy is not nearly as effective in treating cancer if the patient smokes because smoking affects many biological systems. Smoking even two or three cigarettes a day can adversely affect the body. Thus, smokers with cancer are also more likely to die from noncancer causes, such as a heart attack, stroke, or pneumonia.

Smoking also can continue to increase a patient's chances of getting a second cancer, even if a patient has been cured from the first. More than one cancer survivor has lived through one cancer only to die of a second. And it is not only smoking-related cancers that are affected. Quitting smoking will make treatment more effective for any cancer, not just for lung cancer. Also, remember that for some unknown reason, you developed this cancer, not your neighbor. For some reason, your body possibly had some environmental exposure or underlying genetic weakness that led you to get the disease. Because you still have this weakness, you have a higher risk of getting another cancer. Smoking increases this risk even further. While other causes exist and may increase your risk level modestly by 25 to 50 percent, smoking increases your cancer risk far more dramatically by perhaps as many as several thousand percent.

Nothing tells an oncologist that a patient isn't really committed to getting better than when a patient becomes irritated when asked about smoking. Don't become defensive when an oncologist constantly asks about your cigarette smoking. He cares. He's trying. He wants you to stop.

Be cooperative. Ask what works best. It is not unusual for a smoker to have a difficult time quitting. Persist. Try again. It may take months and months to quit. Combinations of medications are sometimes needed. You might need both a medication to cut your drive to smoke and also a patch, gum, or inhaler to replace your nicotine. See which ones work best. Continued close attention and monitoring, and even admonishment, are essential if a smoker is going to stay off of tobacco.

FAMILY SMOKERS

It is particularly hard to quit when family members and friends continue to smoke. It is little help to the patient when these smokers offer to go outside or elsewhere to smoke. The simple fact is that a cancer patient should not be around any smokers at any time. Patients can smell the odor of cigarettes on others even if they are not smoking at that time. These may tempt them to start again. By asking others to stop as well, the experience is shared. Everyone's efforts to quit will be inspirational to one another. They can share stories about what works best to kill the desire for nicotine. They will also have their own little support group. They did offer to help, didn't they?

Joe: Like Father, Like Son

Joe was a 77-year-old lung cancer patient who was luckily cured of both his first and second lung cancers by surgery. He had part of both his right and left lungs removed to treat his cancer. Still he smoked. When I had a serious discussion about the need to quit, his son Dan agreed. He began to chastise his dad about his continued smoking. Later, I had the opportunity to observe both of them drive out of the parking lot. Before they left the lot, BOTH Joe and his son Dan lit up and were smoking! Obviously both were at high risk of developing cancer, and neither had yet learned the importance of quitting. The high risk that both may have shared was the result of a possible inherited tendency toward the cancer, compounded by the smoking. They couldn't change the inherited tendency, but they could have stopped the smoking.

Even though it is very difficult for many to quit smoking, it is ultimately under the patient's control. Having care close to home is also important.

PROXIMITY/AVAILABILITY

Another way to increase your chances of successful treatment is to have a team of physicians who know your condition close by. Even if part of the care is at a facility distant from home, patients still need physicians nearby. Emergencies occur. Most of life will be spent close to home. If local physicians aren't aware of initial procedures done elsewhere, they may not want to step into cases if there are complications from another physicians' procedures. Among some doctors, this situation is known as Frankenstein's Law. In other words, "You created this monster. You deal with it." It may sound harsh, but many physicians justifiably fear assuming someone else's potential liability. To avoid this situation, good communication among all doctors early in a case is best.

For example, if a bladder catheter was inserted during a prostate surgery in a different city, a local urologist can't step in unaware to fix a complication. He wasn't there at the initial procedure. If the first physician did something that could lead to a lawsuit, the second physician might be dragged into the legal case. The second urologist may not want to help because he would be accepting the liability of another person's work. He also would not necessarily be paid. Some physicians may occasionally agree to treat such a case, largely for benevolent reasons, but this cannot be assumed. Good communication between physicians helps, but it is not always done. Paying physicians for having a dialog would probably help the situation, although it is not yet done.

Other reasons exist to have a good relationship with nearby doctors. A physician of a different specialty at home might be needed as well. A good relationship with a local oncologist will help facilitate urgent complex care. Without this, patients are at the mercy of the Emergency Room and whichever physician is on call that evening. Emergent care at home will be much easier to facilitate with these established local relationships.

BRING A FAMILY MEMBER OR FRIEND

It is essential to bring a companion to at least the first consultation. A family member or a friend will be able to listen to the explanation of the cancer and the upcoming surgery or therapy in a more detached manner than the patient. The physician will have greater respect for a patient who has the wisdom to bring another person. He will usually pay more attention when an adult child is present. Explanations are more detailed. Questions are asked for and then answered.

An honesty checkup is seconded by having someone else there. The patient may have forgotten about an event or symptom. For example, people will at times fail to mention that they fell. They think that since the injury was slight, no mention is needed. Actually it is important for your oncologist to explore falling. Did you fall because of a sudden drop in blood pressure from dehydration? Or was it because the nerves surrounding the blood vessels were damaged from chemotherapy? Maybe you had a heart rhythm abnormality? This will hopefully prevent a more serious injury.

At some time during treatment, the patient should introduce his or her adult children to the oncologist. Although it is important to remember that the patient is in charge, children are important family members, whose input generally should be respected. If there is discord within the family as to the extent or type of treatment, it is best to keep all of these issues in the open. Thus, your oncologist will not receive an unpleasant surprise when an upset family member calls with concerns. Introducing a spouse or adult child to the oncologist helps solidify a relationship that will become important if the patient becomes too ill to make decisions. Many times, patients name family members in their durable powers of attorney for health care decisions.

Those patients who face the challenge of going through this journey without families often arrive with more advanced cancers and late complications. It is challenging to try to hire someone to help with this. Families and friends are flexible and compassionate, while employed people can change jobs often and may or may not become the shoulder to lean on that a patient needs. Other organizations, such as volunteers involved with veterans or senior organizations, may help with companion programs.

TREAT PHOBIAS, DENTAL PROBLEMS, ARTHRITIS, AND OTHER DISEASES

It is important for the patient to prepare for cancer treatment. If someone arrives with a litany of other untreated medical problems, it makes care more difficult. Patients may still have an unfinished procedure that they delayed because of family emergencies, Christmas bills, or a job layoff. Dental procedures, treatment for cataracts, arthritis, or hips needing replacement are all problems that people often put off. Some patients use these as shields to protect them from treatment in case surgery or chemotherapy is discussed. This is a form of denial where you hope that when you have other medical priorities, you can justifiably delay cancer treatment or even believe that the cancer will stop growing. "Oh no, I can't get my breast cancer treated. I need to have my teeth done." Or "I couldn't possibly have lung surgery. I need my cataracts fixed."

Those who procrastinate may find themselves needing to do all of these things at once. Patients need to prioritize their medical care. It is unwise to put off lung cancer surgery one month to have a cataract taken out. On the other hand, a serious heart, blood vessel, or long problem should be addressed first. Your oncologists will help you determine the proper sequence of treatment. Listen to her.

A slight twist on this self-defeating theme is if a patient harbors neurosis or other problems that will limit treatment. "I can't get an MRI done because I have claustrophobia," is an all-too common complaint. Few patients have ever said the more appropriate, "I don't think I can get one now, but I'll work with a therapist on relaxation techniques so I may be able to do one later." The first step is to try to recognize what is obstructing treatment. If a patient has other legitimate medical problems, he should ask how to overcome rather than surrender to them.

EXPLAIN CLEARLY

Speak clearly. For many members of the oncologist community, English is not their first language. Simple phrases, such as: "I've been better," said in response to: "How are you?" could be misleading. *I've been better,* sounds like you are improving. As all of us know the true meaning is quite the opposite. By saying: "I feel bad," the chance of a misunderstanding is removed. Other examples are also easy to find. When asked about pain, many patients will say, "Oh, it's nothing that I can't handle." An oncologist is not trying to measure pain tolerance or see if can be ignored. He's trying to ascertain if it is improving or not. "It's still present, but better" is a more useful response, as is "It's worse, especially when I move." By speaking and complaining more simply and directly, you prevent misunderstandings. By carefully describing symptoms, an oncologist can better understand a condition. Keep notes.

The patient who says, "Oh it's nothing I can't handle," is actually giving the oncologist an important clue as to her approach to the cancer and pain. She is trying to be stoic and put up with it. If she admits that the pain might be worsening, she is admitting that the cancer might be spreading and is worried that the physician might get a clue as to how bad she is feeling. She is actually trying to mislead him into helping her to deny worsening pain. Admit what is going on. Honesty works.

SHOW UP

Many important clues to a patient's condition become apparent during a physical exam. If you are sick, try to avoid the temptation to have the oncologist merely call in a medication for you. Often this is a bad idea. Many offices overuse telephone medicine. At times, the physician has only a tangential knowledge about the complaint. In addition, patient description are often incomplete and don't include all of the relevant information. It's easy to confuse a cold with influenza, pneumonia, or worse. Many times, the most important part of the examination is for the physician to eyeball the patient. By showing up and being seen, you greatly increase your oncologist's knowledge of the immediate problem.

After the office is closed, patients are often referred to the emergency room for evaluation. It is common for people to dread and curse the emergency room. The long wait on an uncomfortable gurney when someone is sick makes this feeling understandable. But emergency rooms are essential for care. They provide a tremendously useful service. At any time of day, you can be seen by a physician anywhere in the country who is usually very thorough and conscientious. Extensive testing, including appropriate lab, X-ray, and CAT scans, can be done and interpreted immediately. Amazing. They'll even pick you up at home if you're too sick.

You should avoid the tendency to think of the emergency room as the last resort. You don't have to pass out first or wait until you are nearly dead to go there. It is better to go to the emergency room and be checked out than to wait and arrive in respiratory, cardiac, or kidney failure. If in doubt, go and get checked out. If you can't make it to the ER, call 911. In my experience, far more patients avoid the emergency room than abuse it for trivial reasons. It is rare that a patient's ER visit is denied by insurance. You're never too sick to go to the doctor. It is also important to make sure that your records are forwarded to your oncologist on the next business day.

THE CURSE OF THE SELF-EMPLOYED

Dan owned his own cleaning service. He had been the third of eight children born to a fanatically clean dairy farmer. The hard work and cleaning habits learned from his family's dairy farm business had served him well in making his own business very successful. When he developed a large throat cancer, I warned him about what I called "the curse of the self-employed." He gradually understood, all too well, what I meant. He was accustomed to making his business a priority. He would answer calls late into the night every night. If an employee failed him in some way, he would take over himself.

All of these attributes that made him a great small business owner worked against him when he was sick. Later when he was very ill and needed to stay later in the clinic for extra treatments, he would think twice when torn by a work commitment. He would not refuse when an admission to the hospital was strongly recommended, however. Instead, he understood how important it was to put his health first.

Many self-employed business owners have terrible records of taking care of their own health. They will arrange regular check-ups for their business trucks or computers, but not for themselves. Years go by with no health care at all. They fail to develop knowledge of their own body, of exercise, of how to be a patient, and of how to take care of themselves. An employee of a business with great benefits will take advantage of a personal day off to get a routine check-up, but the small business owner will not. Instead, he sees only lost revenue from a closed shop.

You need to try to avoid this temptation and instead prioritize *you*. Your health is first. Routine maintenance is not only for your car.

Many high-level corporate employees will also continue their dedication to work to the detriment of their health. If you don't have a back-up plan for yourself at work, make one. Here is where redundancy in your job position is good. Try to avoid the temptation to use work as an excuse to not get the treatment you deserve.

FOCUS ON YOU

This is a good transition into ways to focus on yourself. If patients learn how to gain acceptance of their diseases and the correct role of work in their lives, they can begin to focus on THEMSELVES. If they allow it, they will learn a great deal about who they are from the process. Many ways exist to help. Local support groups and cancer centers may have enlightening programs. Patients might consider seeing a psychologist merely to gain insight into how to handle such a crisis. Many patients are better able to relax during a test when they have learned biofeedback or other relaxation methods. By becoming more familiar with their own bodies and minds, patients help their oncologists by avoiding the creation of unnecessary obstacles.

NUTRITION/WEIGHT LOSS/DIETARY SUPPLEMENTS

Good nutrition will help tremendously in the fight against cancer, as a huge part of the effort is maintaining a stable weight and good eating habits. Patients will find many avenues of advice about the proper use of vitamins and supplements. You could also see a dietician, especially if you also have diabetes. Dieticians may be helpful in customizing a diet for you. For example, patients at risk for bowel blockage, such as women with ovarian cancer, may need to avoid hard-to-digest food, such as steak or the insides of oranges. Because these foods may not get fully digested, they can contribute to an obstruction. Patients with stomach surgery might need to avoid carbohydrates to keep from having dumping syndrome, in which diarrhea follows a high carbohydrate meal. Patients who have had throat radiation therapy may need to have thickeners added to their liquids to prevent aspiration. Even if it is an out-of-pocket expense, dieticians and proper nutrition are worth the money.

Many cancers will cause weight loss by producing hormones. By keeping weight stable, the body can better handle the stresses of both the cancer and the treatments. The loss of more than 10 percent of a patient's usual weight contributes to a bad prognosis. Even if you are overweight at the outset of the illness, it is important to keep weight stable. Medications that induce hunger and increase weight gain are useful. These medications can be combined with nutritional supplements to help keep body weight stable. Ask your oncologist to help select the correct dietary supplement. Generally, patients are advised to avoid preparations that contain excessive salt or others that can cause bowel changes.

Often, cancer patients complain about food tasting bad. There are tricks to help food taste better so that you'll eat more. First, treat any yeast or viral infection. If food leaves a metallic taste in the mouth, try using plasticware instead of normal silverware. Other times, varying the spices on food may help a patient regain some appetite.

Diabetes is a common complication caused by cancers or their treatment. The way that a body handles sugar is often temporarily affected by medications such as steroids. Weight loss and cancers in or near the pancreas can also wreak havoc with blood sugars. See a trained dietician. This will greatly improve the chances of keeping weight stable, too.

The minerals iron and magnesium and vitamins B12 and D are common nutritional deficiencies found in many cancer patients. Many who have colon cancer are low in iron and have slowly lost iron for years. Most women are also substantially low on iron from years of having menstrual periods. Taking iron supplements will help the healing process after surgery and during radiation therapy. It will also help increase a patient's energy level and may lower the chance of an allergic-type reaction to chemotherapy. Ask your oncologist to check iron levels. Patients very low in iron have a curious tendency to crave ice chewing—particularly soft ice.

Often older women don't have a good level of vitamin D, so this should be checked and addressed to help prevent bone fractures and loss of height. Spinal compression fractures and hip fractures are common complications of cancer treatment. By taking calcium and vitamin D, patients help to prevent these painful complications.

HYGIENE

A seldom discussed and sometimes uncomfortable subject is hygiene. Meticulous attention to it will help prevent wound infection. Staph is a skin bacterium that lives on many of us. Problems can be caused by these bugs. By washing yourself with antibacterial soaps before any surgical procedure, you may prevent infections. By going into surgery without having done this you greatly increase your chances of infection complications. Staph can also reside in the nasal area. Many facilities are routinely checking for this now. Antibiotic cream may be prescribed for use in this area before surgery.

Other complications can also occur without proper attention to hygiene. Dental care is essential. Your teeth should be professionally cleaned on a regular basis in addition to daily brushing and flossing at home. If your maintain good teeth and gums, you dramatically improve your chance of not having various health problems. Patients who pay this much attention to their health seem to have fewer infections.

EXERCISE

Exercise is another key to improving the your chances of survival. Your health can be affected when you are in bed for long periods of time. Bedsores, skin breakdown, pneumonias, blood clots, and depression are all affected by a lack of exercise. You can prevent many complications by exercising. For example, walking and exercise can help prevent deep vein thrombosis (or leg blood clots), lung blood clots, pneumonias, and other infections. Pushing oneself to walk every day, even when you are very weak, is crucial. Any walking will always help. Ask a friend for support if you need it.

Long-term goals for exercising should include aerobic exercising and light weightlifting under supervision. With the help of a trainer, when approved by an oncologist, these activities will aid patients in preventing long-term complications, such as bone loss and osteoporosis. Ask your bones to be strong by exercising. Taking a bone pill won't do it by itself.

Cancer patients shouldn't wear themselves out thinking of excuses why they shouldn't exercise. The goal is to find the solutions to help survive. If knees hurt when walking, try walking in water. If it's too cold outside, take the laundry off the treadmill and use that. It may be safest to work out in a fitness facility where there are others nearby to help.

FOLLOW-UP VISITS/PERIODIC TESTS

Routine follow-up visits with an oncologist are essential. Most cancer patients gain from seeing an oncologist in addition to seeing a family physician and surgeon. Oncologists are tuned into complications that can occur from previous treatments. They're are also astute at looking for second and even third cancers that may develop.

Keep in mind that the tests done at a follow-up visit don't tell the physician all he needs to know. Most of the information that he gets is as a result of the interview at the time of the visit. She relies on patient input. Has weight been lost? Is there any new back pain? Or a new breast lump? These follow-up visits are key to helping prevent future problems. Don't miss them.

EMPOWER YOURSELF

Details matter. Don't fall into the "whatever" attitude. Patients need to work on helping themselves survive. This starts by getting past grief and depression, giving up harmful addictions, and knowing the body—and getting to the doctor at the right time. Of all the patients I've seen, the ones who do best are the ones who have a proactive attitude, not a passive one.

WHAT'S NEXT

The patient has been treated. He or she feels better and is slowly coming back. The next chapter will show how to deal with some of the most important concerns at this new stage, as patients return to travel, work, and sex.

Chapter 11

Back to Your Life

When to Say "Yes" to Travel, Work, Exercise, and Sex

It is encouraging to resume the routine of everyday life. Getting back to work, relaxation, family, relationships, and personal time is refreshing. There is something very reassuring about performing what were once mundane activities. Yes, cancer is still real, and yes, patients are being inconvenienced by labs, scans, treatments, and clinic appointments, but normal is good.

One primary goal of treatment, in addition to ensuring survival, is to allow the patient to return to everyday life. This includes gardening, family gatherings, holidays, camping trips, romantic and intimate evenings, work, and all the rest of your life. Without these activities, patients lose the motivation to keep trying. But finding the correct balance between personal time and treatment responsibilities is difficult. Enjoying fun time with your family is great, but jeopardizing your health is not.

There is an unwritten contract between a cancer patient and the oncologist. When the physician agrees to the treatment with powerful chemotherapy drugs, he is relying on the person with whom he is working. He assumes that you bring a certain amount of responsibility and common sense to the table. You need to quickly notify the correct person when you are ill or in trouble. Going to see your family for a short visit a few hours away makes sense. Complicated travel for a protracted time may not.

Louis: His Job Was His Life

Louis was a 60-year-old man who was committed to his work. He enjoyed being an important member of the company by team driving for a family business. In fact, he had been its key driver for 27 years. One Sunday he felt ill, developing a low-grade temperature, nausea, weakness, and lightheadedness. By the next day, he was feeling slightly better and hoped to drive on Tuesday. Unfortunately, the job took him several states away. By the end of the week, he was hospitalized in intensive care. He had septic shock (a bloodstream infection that mimics flu-like symptoms and will cause death in five or six days if untreated). The risk of infections is particularly high in cancer patients with compromised immune systems. Cancer patients may also not appreciate that infections may be present with minimal symptoms, such as only mild chills and a low-grade temperature.

The dedication that Louis had for his job was admirable but not worth risking his life for. It didn't make sense.

WORK

The mutual goal of the patient and oncology team is to get a person back to work—safely. Whether he or she holds a formal job or not, resuming work is essential. It improves self-worth and helps ward off depression. When a person, any person, contributes to the community, he or she feels better and productive and becomes more tolerant of allowing others to help them. By being productive, a person improves his or her chances of long-term survival. Most patients can reasonably hope to return to work at least part-time during their cancer treatments.

Having an employer who is flexible and understanding is essential. Bosses who have a personal history of cancer in their families are far more compassionate.

WORK ENVIRONMENTS

It is good to know that certain situations can lead to problems. Louis, our worker who drove several states away for his job above, is an example of someone who may need to consider a safer work environment. Jobs where you work heavy machinery or drive for long distances may not be the best for cancer patients. Part of the reason is that many treatments can cause fatigue or disrupt sleep routines. Also, cancer patients are at high risk for blood clots known as DVTs, or deep vein thromboses. Blood clots such as these can cause several problems. In the immediate area where they develop, such as the legs, pain or edema occurs. More serious problems can occur when these clots move, such as when one moves to your lungs causing a pulmonary embolus. Clots develop more easily when cancer causes your body's elaborately controlled system of bleeding and clotting to become mixed up.

For someone with cancer, driving for more than an hour or two causes blood pools in the legs and may promote the development of clots. Sudden onset of shortness of breath and chest pain that occurs after starting to walk are signs that the clots have moved to the lungs, a potentially fatal complication. Other work environments that may be less than ideal are places that are likely to be too hot or cold. The weight loss and nerve damage that is caused by cancer and its treatments make it harder for the body to adjust to temperature extremes.

CLEAN WORK ENVIRONMENT

Work environments need to be clean, safe, and not put the patient at risk for more problems. Jobs where you might acquire an infection, such as manual labor or farm work, can be dangerous. Any environment that is dirty or where you are exposed to animal or human waste can be a problem. Likewise, by working around others with infections, such as in a nursing home, cancer patients put themselves at too high a risk. They should ask to be reassigned to avoid the acutely ill.

As usual, people who work for themselves might easily put themselves at risk. Examples are when a self-employed roofer with numb feet thinks he can still navigate the steep pitch of a roof and falls. Because many self-employed people don't have adequate disability insurance, they push their luck. Another example is a farmer who continues to work around farm animals and gets infections related to animal waste. If working involves unclean situations, such as the ones I've described, it's probably best to notify an oncologist. By telling physicians of a patient's concerns, treatments can be adapted to help lower the chances of infections.

One example of how treatments can be adapted is through the use of a port, which is a permanent, central-line intravenous catheter hidden under the skin. Two types of permanently implanted central venous catheters are used. One called a port is completely under the skin and thereby protected from infection by your skin. The chance of infections is lower with these catheters than with the other central-line catheter that hangs loosely out of the body. These catheters still leave the patient susceptible to infection through the skin.

Patients should also consider environmental exposures at work. Some significant ones include sun, chemicals such as herbicides or other carcinogens, and radiation. Radiation exposure may occur in the energy, medical and, possibly, airline industries. Many other work-related issues include excess noise, stress, shift work, and certain odors.

LIFTING

No matter who you are, be wary about lifting or moving heavy objects at work. Cancer patients, however, are at an increased risk of bone fractures for several reasons. These include direct destruction of the bones from cancer. In addition, hormone and radiation treatments can accelerate osteoporosis leading to fractures. Many cancer patients are elderly and have already developed osteoporosis. Lifting heavy or awkward objects might lead to painful and disabling hip and spine fractures. Such objects include suitcases and lawnmowers. It may also mean lighter but important wiggly objects such as babies. Compression fractures of the spine occur frequently and can cause a great deal of pain and disability. Swinging an axe, lifting a lawnmower, and moving a desk are examples of ways in which patients have fractured their spines. It is usually better to let things fall rather than break bones.

HYDRATION

Consuming lots of water can be essential after being treated for cancer. Throat radiation or weak blood pressure, for example, make adequate hydration a must. Depending on the work environment, patients may need extra time for water and bathroom breaks. Others have had to readjust their work environment to be closer to the bathroom. They'll definitely need extra time for breaks if they've had radiation to the pelvis. Some patients need frequent sips of water to replace the normal saliva that they lost and may take to wearing water backpacks like skiers or the members of the military.

Several key observations let you determine if you are adequately hydrated. Concentrated or dark urine may be as sign that you are becoming dehydrated. It is important to keep up an adequate amount of urine as well. You shouldn't go the entire day without relieving yourself. Other signs of dehydration are lightheadedness, dizziness, or passing out. It never fails to surprise me that some patients will actually try to control diarrhea by not drinking. This ensures dehydration, as you are not drinking enough to keep up with your body's fluid losses.

Diarrhea may be controlled with a variety of medications that are available without prescription. It is important, however, to inform your oncologist of the severity of the diarrhea, as it may be a sign of a several types of bowel infections. If not addressed, these infections have been known to become chronic, serious, and potentially fatal. Dealing with chronic diarrhea is important. It may also be caused by a number of cancer or precancer conditions. Several chemotherapy drugs and radiation therapy are also common causes of diarrhea.

CRITICAL PERSONNEL

In thinking about work arrangements, cancer patients need to consider if their presence in the office is critical. Being the only one who can do a particular job is dangerous in terms of health. Some of the patients who fit in this category are the self-employed and those with special skills. At one time or another, because they didn't have a backup person to call, people in these professions have stayed on the job until they passed out or worse.

Avoiding this is best. The body can only handle so much stress and illness. When people feel so committed to a job that they won't leave even if they are acutely ill, they need to discuss matters with their bosses. Redundancy is good. Get a deputy—someone at work who is able to take over when you must go. Numerous patients have stayed on the job despite life threatening symptoms of infections or bleeding out of duty. Don't be afraid to leave your post at work. Lives are worth it.

TRAVEL

With cancer, even travel is complicated. Many of us expect to be able to board a jet plane and travel to other parts of the country at a moment's notice. For the cancer patient, travel is risky.

keep their fertility, many still do. Other options, including adoption are also very real. By bringing these concerns to your oncologist, you improve your odds of being able to have children.

Bill: Prioritizing Intimacy

Bill, a slightly forgetful and aging policeman, was being treated for a penile cancer. His wife of 60 years answered most of the questions. After numerous consultations with radiation oncologists and surgeons, Bill was unable to bring himself to agree to the recommended "amputation" surgery or the similarly unacceptable radiation. Chemotherapy was of marginal benefit as the amount of treatment he was able to tolerate only held his disease stable. One day, his wife sheepishly asked if it were safe for them to have marital relations. I advised them about safe methods and medications to help. Later when asked if it worked, she remarked that they hadn't had the energy yet, but they had hope.

It is every individual's right to prioritize intimacy over ultimate survival. Don't be embarrassed to ask.

Zach: Spicing Up a Sterile Environment

Zach was a well-built 35-year-old married man with an aggressive lung cancer. The treatment of his disease resulted in endless frustrating hospitalizations over many months. Lucky for him, Lizzie, his devoted wife, always seemed to be by his side. She kept up his spirits, and they were inseparable. Their little known secret was a game *exploring* unused sections of the hospital late at night and on weekends for fun and intimacy. They would also often leave a little sign that they had been there. Their secret game added some excitement to the stale hospital environment.

Even though some of the patients in these stories had challenging times and a few even passed away, they enjoyed the warmth, love, and support from the physical intimacy flowing from their relationships. It's obvious to me that this love and intimacy supported them and their spouses. Memories of the bonding of these times will be treasured by you and your survivors.

Ralph and Lilly: Bonding Through Prayer and Intimacy

Ralph was a very religious man devoted to his family and wife. He had quite a few children. When his cancer treatment required a protracted hospital stay at a specialized surgical center far from home, the entire clan went. Between attending to his kids, work duties, and his medical care, there was little time for bonding with his wife. But undeterred, every day, his wife Lilly would conspire with the local minister to send the kids to the playground, place a PRAYING—DO NOT DISTURB sign on the door, and spend a half hour of quality intimate time with her husband. These times together gave Ralph something to look forward to each day despite many monotonous and uncomfortable hours.

You shouldn't feel any shame or embarrassment in arranging space for intimacy with your partner. Be creative. Be fun. Be bold. Be loved.

EMPOWER YOURSELF

Remember that everyday activities help you cope with the trauma and shock of your cancer diagnosis. It is great to be ambitious and want to travel, work, exercise, and be intimate, but be safe and be sure it makes sense. These activities define who you are. Don't get caught up in being a full-time patient. Play.

WHAT'S NEXT

How does a cancer patient continue once they've been diagnosed? The supportive care insights that follow won't be found in any book. They are based on my experience.

Chapter 12

Supportive Care Insights
How to Better Tolerate Treatment

F

ew patients willingly agree to therapy that has intolerable side effects. Many unwittingly expect treatments to be ineffective unless accompanied by substantial amounts of nausea, vomiting, and hair loss. Often patients give up on the opportunity for considering cancer treatment without appreciating that many treatments can be made far more tolerable. With close attention to details and good communication with the oncology office, these and many other dreaded side effects become minor, not major, complaints. Much of the common wisdom surrounding side effects doesn't apply.

If you are nauseated several days after chemotherapy, should nausea medication be taken or will this actually worsen the problem? Should a laxative be taken instead?

If you have diarrhea, should you take an over the counter medication or is it severe enough to tell your oncologist?

What are the symptoms of an infection from a permanent intravenous catheter?

How can you and your oncologist work together to help prevent bone weakening and fractures?

I don't feel like eating and I'm nauseated. Do I really need to move my bowels daily?

These and many other questions may seem too trivial to bother the oncologist with, but they are crucial to your experience. If you don't know

145

how to tolerate your treatment, you won't continue them. Most patients are surprised to learn by experience that chemotherapy treatments become unexpectedly easier to tolerate as time passes. Being familiar with how your body reacts will help you know how to prevent side effects. Take a laxative when you know that you will get constipated. Take acetaminophen when you know that a certain chemotherapy drug will give you a temperature.

IV (INTRAVENOUS) ACCESS CATHETERS

Many cancer patients require IV access catheters for antibiotics, nutrition, chemotherapy, hydration, nausea, and other medications. As discussed, these catheters are called ports or central lines and are used for faster access of IV drugs. Several options exist, including devices inserted under the skin as well as those with tubes left dangling outside. In our experience, the catheters left under the skin appear safer and have a lower chance for infections. Usually these are placed by an experienced surgeon in the upper chest wall of the patient. Several complications can occur. One is a pneumothorax, or air trapped in the chest outside the lung, resulting in a deflated lung (dropping a lung). Other complications include bleeding at the site. Some of the common long-term risks include infections, as well as blood clots in the veins in which these catheters run. Only people experienced with these devices should be using or accessing them. When inexperienced staff or people without proper supplies try to utilize them, it can lead to risks. Both infections and blood clots can be challenging to discover. Blood clots show up as pain or a vague discomfort in the chest or as swelling of the arm nearest to the catheter. An ultrasound or CAT scan may help to diagnose these clots. Treatment may include removal of the catheter or use of blood thinners either by mouth or as an injection. Newer blood thinning agents, such as Lovenox (enoxaparin), Arixtra (fondaparinux), Fragmen (dalteparin), and Innohep (tinzaparin) have helped to permit many patients with blood clots in the veins to be treated as outpatients. Also other drugs, such as alteplase, are able to actually dissolve blood clots found within the catheters.

The symptoms for infections in indwelling catheters are vague and may include low grade temperatures, chills, and sweats. These symptoms may go on for weeks or longer. One day the patient may feel only slightly weak; the next day, he or she may have serious chills, a temperature, and low blood pressure from a possible bloodstream infection. The catheter needs to be flushed at intervals prescribed by the attending physician. As soon as possible, remove the catheter to reduce the risks of infection, clots, and other complications. If a patient's plans include travel, he or she may need to relay them to the oncologist to better facilitate catheter care and infection and clot prevention while away.

Joe and Jack: A Tale of Two Catheters

Joe, age 66, was treated for a lung cancer several years before. He had chemotherapy a year previously and still had a port-type catheter in his chest. While his follow-up visits had been okay and his cancer did not return, he refused to have the port removed. (Later he confessed that he quietly worried that if his chest port was removed, his cancer would return.) He developed a fever one weekend, but thought it was from a chest cold. Despite not feeling 100 percent, he went to work driving his truck several states away. Two days later in a distant state, he developed fevers, chills, and weakness; he went to the emergency room. Septic, with a blood stream infection, he was soon in the intensive care unit. He barely survived. In a month, after a protracted hospital stay, he returned home to convalescence. The reason for his infections was a slowly developing staph infection in the port in his chest. Had the port been removed, he may not have become ill.

Jack, age 55, with non-Hodgkin's lymphoma, spent Christmas in a distant city visiting his family. He was on a month-long break from his chemotherapy; his chest catheter was functioning just fine and was not hurting or draining. His wife called back home to us, asking if the 101.5 temperature meant that he needed to be seen in the emergency room. Although he balked at going, we insisted that he be checked out. He claimed that he hoped it was a cold.

While Jack may indeed have a cold, when you have a semipermanent central-line catheter, it makes sense to pay close attention to any signs of infection. The staph infections that are common in these catheters can easily masquerade as other common infections and maladies.

BOWEL TROUBLES

In medical school I learned the insensitive wisdom that if I were ever in a room with a patient and needed time to think, I could stall by asking the patient about his bowels. Troubles with keeping a system regular can be very serious. Numerous aspects of cancer and its treatment can cause sluggish bowels, which in turn may cause a lot of discomfort and pain. It can also affect quality of life and the ability to continue treatment. One small example is when patients relay that they find themselves without any nausea for the first day or two after chemotherapy, but have troubles on day two or three. They are actually suffering from nausea and abdominal discomfort due to lazy bowel troubles (caused by the nausea medications given in the vein along with the chemotherapy medication). Lazy bowel, or ileus in medical terms, is when drugs, surgery, or immobility cause bowels to bind up and not move as well as they should. Patients feel much better, have less nausea. and have less pain if they are regular.

CONSTIPATION

Pain medications, nausea medications, inactivity, and certain chemotherapy drugs are some of the common causes of constipation. All narcotic drugs, however, regardless of whether they are given through the IV or by mouth, cause severe constipation. It is expected that most all of our patients need the "poop talk" as they start on treatments. Therefore, plan on taking laxatives at the start when taking any narcotic (*not* after someone hasn't pooped for three days). If more pain medication is prescribed, more laxatives should be taken. Certain oral iron medications, as well as heart medications known as calcium channel blockers, also cause constipation. Rarely are patients alerted to these facts. Inactivity is a biggie when it comes to bowels. Simple walking can help this (walking also helps prevent blood clots, pneumonias, and other problems). A good rule of thumb is to try to have one or two normal bowl movements per day. Ask doctors for advice if it has been more than three days since a patient has gone to the bathroom. Don't use enemas or suppositories if there is a low blood count or if surgery on the rectum is needed (unless you're physician is notified). Don't assume that all abdominal pain is the result of cancer or even surgery. If there is abdominal pain—and there hasn't been a BM in several days—consider trying a laxative before assuming it is cancer pain.

Diarrhea

A common complication of colon surgery, intestinal radiation therapy, and of various medications is diarrhea. Common medications include any type of magnesium product, certain chemotherapy drugs, and certain antibiotics. Another frequent cause of diarrhea is a bowel infection caused by changes in intestinal flora because of antibiotics and other stresses. It's helpful to restore the normal bowel flora with yogurt and other similar preparations that contain live cultures. Regardless of the cause of diarrhea, it is important to stay well hydrated. On many occasions I have had patients arrive lightheaded, weak, and dehydrated after bouts of severe diarrhea. Some have died from this alone. Others have become critically ill, developed renal failure, or even died of dehydration at home because they were too embarrassed about having an accident on the way to the clinic or hospital. Some signs of dehydration are lightheadedness, dizziness when standing, a general feeling of weakness, or poor urine output.

The infection that causes diarrhea in cancer patients is commonly known as C. Diff, which is short for clostridium difficile. The bug is an overgrowth normally contained by other bugs in intestinal flora. When stress or antibiotics change the normal makeup inside you, diarrhea ensues. It can be treated a number of ways, with a combination of yogurt, antibiotics, and fiber preparations. Medications used to slow the bowels are not used here. This type of bowel infection is very common but easily overlooked. It can complicate another frequent cause of diarrhea, which is radiation injury. At times both patients and physicians will assume that cancer treatments, such as radiation therapy and chemotherapy, are the only cause of the patient's diarrhea. However, it is not unusual for diarrhea to have several causes. You might have diarrhea because of chemotherapy and a c. diff infection. Unless both causes are treated, the diarrhea won't go away. It should not be assumed that there is only one cause of a problem.

IRON, MAGNESIUM, POTASSIUM

Many cancer patients are critically low on iron, whether they are women or men. Many colon cancer patients have such low iron reserves that they are anemic. They can lose iron by bleeding—it's the only way. Most of the time this blood loss occurs slowly in imperceptible ways through the intestine. Regular menstrual periods in women, obviously, are another cause of serious blood loss. Another frequent cause of blood loss is radiation injury to the rectum. Regardless of the manner in which the blood is lost, the complications still occur. By restoring normal iron levels through supplements—and good diet, more rapid recovery from surgeries and other stresses can be promoted. People who have their iron levels restored also feel stronger.

Magnesium and other trace electrolytes are also key to helping the body tolerate cancer and its treatment. Certain chemotherapy drugs can cause a person to become depleted in magnesium. The body will have a difficult time restoring normal calcium balance unless magnesium levels are restored. Further, patients may have fewer severe reactions to certain chemotherapy agents if magnesium levels are normal.

Potassium is an important chemical in the body. Many drugs and medical conditions will deplete the patient of it. These include vomiting, diarrhea, diuretics, and other medications. Developing kidney failure will cause potassium to become critically high. However, it can be replaced most effectively by taking an oral supplement. IV potassium is slow and inefficient. When potassium is abnormal, the heart tends to have trouble staying in a normal rhythm. Keeping potassium in range helps to avoid this and the patient stays stronger.

EDEMA (OR SWELLING)

Arms, legs, and other body parts can become markedly swollen when there is cancer. In many instances this is the result of poor nutrition and is directly related to a body protein named albumin. It's is called a carrier protein, which means many drugs or hormones are bound or stuck to it when they travel through the blood. A good measure of nutrition is when the body is busy making the normal amount of albumin, as it is albumin that will prevent swelling, or edema, of the feet. After substantial weight loss because of cancer, the body no longer makes an adequate amount of the protein. As a result, tissue fluids in the extremities leaking out, thereby causing edema. Other reasons for edema include poor kidney function, excessive salt intake, and obstructions to blood return caused by cancer or medical devices.

Swelling can be helped by a variety of measures. Some involve taking dietary supplements or limiting salt intake. Other aids are elevating the legs and wearing tight stockings that compress the legs and thighs. A combination of stockings, massages, limiting salt intake, and prevention works. Exercise, even just walking, will help to prevent edema from developing. Any type of obstruction to blood or tissue fluid (known as lymph fluid) in the back of the abdomen will cause swelling because large groups of swollen lymph nodes in the abdomen will cause swelling in the legs. In addition, filters placed in the blood vessel known as the IVC, or inferior vena cava, will also produce leg edema. Newer filters are being made that are temporary and can be removed if swelling develops. Radiation to the pelvis or legs can be a cause of swelling which is difficult to treat.

NAUSEA AND VOMITING

Expected. Dreaded. The usual. No! Many wrongly expect that for their treatments to work, they must undergo months of nausea and vomiting. These side effects should be very preventable in almost everyone. To prevent nausea and vomiting, many factors must be addressed, including anticipation and anxiety, stomach irritation and gastritis, constipation, and motion sickness, to name a few. The first step toward relieving nausea and vomiting is to rely on prevention. Don't save the best nausea medication for when it's really, really needed. Use it now. First. Many protocols call for using less expensive, less effective nausea medications first, then using the more expensive nausea medication later if you need it. The opposite is sometimes a better technique if the patient is anxious. Then, as confidence is gained, treatments will be better tolerated. At that time, the amount and number of nausea medications can be reduced.

Recovering alcoholics are somehow strangely protected from having much nausea and vomiting. Diabetics, on the other hand, are unusually sensitive to them if caused by chemotherapy. Seeing a primary care physician to try to have better control of diabetes will help.

Overuse of certain nausea medications can paradoxically cause nausea as a result of sluggish bowels. Prescriptions such as ondasetron or granisitron, as well as other drugs, including blood pressure medications can also cause constipation. If there is not a bowel movement for several days, there is a higher chance of having nausea.

Since the early 1990s, new classes of drugs have become available that should be able to control most nausea and vomiting. Even better medications have been approved during the last year or two that control the de-layed nausea that may occur two or three days after your treatments. Emend (Aprepitant), Anzemet (Dolasetron), Kytril (Granisetron), Zofran (Ondansetron) and Aloxi (Palonosetron) are the names of some of these medications.

Treating stomach irritations, such as gastritis, ulcers, and infections, also helps to control nausea and vomiting. Many smokers have chronic stomach irritation that should be treated. Stomach irritations like these are relatively easy to treat, frequently with over-the-counter medications. Gastritis can be alleviated with omeprazole, ranitiding, or similar drugs. Your physician can easily check for bacteria that can aggravate stomach ulcers. If you have such bacteria, antibiotics will be prescribed. Patients who are on oral or intravenous versions of medication known as steroids also develop gastritis. Yet another reason for poor control of nausea and vomiting is when there is a yeast infection of the mouth, throat, or esophagus known as thrush. This infection is easily treated with antifungal liquids that require a prescription.

Anticipation is a large part of nausea and vomiting. Too many people start their chemotherapy treatments expecting to get sick. Notifying an oncologist that there is anxiety about treatments can help him better prepare the patient. Certain medications called anxiolytics are able to treat both anxiety and nausea simultaneously. Biofeedback can also be used to help relieve anxiety. If particularly anxious, ask for reassurance that the best nausea medications be used first rather than saving them in the event that you might get sick.

At times unusual reasons for nausea come into play. One patient had nausea every time she went home from chemotherapy. She was becoming motion sick riding in the back seat of her son's car. It was remedied fairly easily by having her sit in the front seat.

Beth: No Side Effects from Chemo

Beth, a retired school teacher, enjoyed social activities including going to church. When she developed ovarian cancer, she expected that her chemotherapy treatments would be accompanied by extremes of nausea and vomiting. She had also expected the loving support of the friends she grew to know at church. After recovery from her surgery, she hesitantly began her chemotherapy treatments. She was given nausea medications that worked, and she was pleasantly surprised that she tolerated her treatments well. One of her friends at church had a bad experience and became violently ill with her chemotherapy treatments. With good intentions, this church friend reassured Beth each week that the day would come where she would have increasing side effects, including nausea and vomiting, and if she needed help, to call. Each week of her months of therapy the friend repeated her pledge, but Beth never needed help. She never was sick, never vomited. Not once.

Expect to do well. There are lots of great medicines available to prevent nausea. And don't listen to even the most well-meaning naysayers.

BONE PROBLEMS

Many aspects of cancer can cause bone loss and fractures. Medications, radiation treatments, poor nutrition, and cancer itself can all cause bone weakening. By recognizing the bone loss, further decreases can be prevented during healing. Even though good techniques are available to monitor the bone, not everyone is able to benefit from them.

Never assume bones are normal. A DEXA or a bone density scan is a useful tool to help monitor bone loss. Breast and prostate cancer medications are common causes of osteoporosis. Poor nutrition and low levels of vitamin D are other causes. Tremendous numbers of people are affected daily by hip and spine fractures. Many useful drugs and treatments are available to help. Both intravenous and oral drugs can be given along with vitamin D and calcium. For patients with advanced cancer, Aredia (pamidronate) and Zometa (zoledronic acid) are used to prevent bone fractures. By themselves, calcium and vitamin D are useful, but insufficient. Exercise is also key to having healthy bones. Weight resistance exercise taught by a trainer can be directed toward structurally important areas. After obtaining a release from a physician, weight training can strengthen critical bones, including back and hips, over time.

PRIMARY CARE INVOLVEMENT

Depression, blood pressure medication changes, and thyroid issues are some of the reasons primary care physicians should stay involved in a patient's case as cancer treatment begins. Substantial weight loss and appetite changes can affect many aspects of a person's health. A patient may need adjustment in blood pressure or diabetic medications. It is not unusual to notice lightheadedness if blood pressure medications are not adjusted during weight loss. Steroids that are very commonly used in oncology frequently play havoc with blood sugars for several days. Patients will commonly pass out from low blood pressure or low blood sugars when these issues are overlooked.

Dana: Medications

Dana was an overweight 70-year-old man with diabetes, hypertension, heart disease, and a newly diagnosed lung cancer. His small cell lung cancer, however, resulted in a quick 30-pound weight loss. He had been accustomed to always running high blood pressure despite regularly taking several medications.

As he lost weight around the time of his diagnosis, he noticed that he would often become lightheaded and dizzy. Initially he thought nothing of this, but once, after a day's work in his garden late in the spring, he nearly passed out. When he finally reported this, his doctors noticed that his blood pressure would drop substantially when he got up. The dose of blood pressure medication which was appropriate for him before he developed cancer and lost weight was now far too high. By simply adjusting his medications, he was able to reverse the lightheadedness.

Keeping up with your primary care physician can improve your quality of life by keeping a watch on your entire health profile.

Cory: Lowering Thyroid Dose Caused Problems

Cory, a 66-year-old airplane mechanic, developed a throat cancer several years ago. His radiation and chemotherapy treatments were effective, and they resulted in a durable remission. Unfortunately, he also developed a low thyroid condition, which was not unexpected. He went to the emergency room one evening after he had developed a rapid heartbeat. While the emergency room physician was able to treat the cardiac condition easily, he also lowered the thyroid dose substantially. The doctor thought that the thyroid medication had contributed to the rapid heart rate. Cory never thought to recheck the thyroid condition with his family doctor as he was feeling normal. Over time, he developed a very tender abdomen, which brought him to the doctor's office. An X-ray of his abdomen found rather substantial constipation that proved challenging to explain and treat. After a week of tests, it was discovered that his thyroid dose was profoundly underactive. His undertreated thyroid was responsible for his fatigue and for his severe constipation. Keep up with your family physician.

EMPOWER YOURSELF

Details matter. There are ways to tolerate cancer treatment. You can overcome problems such as nausea, vomiting, diarrhea, IV access catheters, and bone loss. By working carefully with the oncologist, as well as the primary care physician, the patient's life can be made far more tolerable.

WHAT'S NEXT

In Chapters 13 and 14, you will learn my from my experience in treating various cancers. From brain tumors to lung to breast to prostate cancer, they all add important nuances to treatment that are important to know.

Chapter 13

Clinical Wisdom
How I Might Do It

If you were diagnosed with breast cancer today, your oncologist would give you the option of a having a mastectomy or a lumpectomy plus radiation therapy. How do you decide?

If you were diagnosed with a throat cancer today, how would you decide between the options of removal of the larynx (voice box) or a combination treatment with chemotherapy and radiation therapy?

How do you improve your chances of recovering from colon cancer surgery without complications?

If your bladder cancer was removed in surgery today, would you know to ask for an opinion with an oncologist when you are told by your other physicians that all you need is close follow-up?

You have developed a colon cancer that has metastasized (or spread) extensively to the liver. Your sigmoid (or lower) colon is nearly obstructed with tumor. Should you see a surgeon to remove the primary cancer in the colon or see an oncologist to start chemotherapy? Or both.

The recommendations that a oncologist gives are based on a combination of clinical wisdom and years of information from research studies. Experience helps him or her judge if treatment should be offered. It also provides the basis for an assessment on whether the cancer patient is too weak or too malnourished to be treated. Perhaps he or she appears tenuous and anxious, or maybe has a preexisting kidney or heart condition.

Over time, it becomes second nature for the oncologist to know if someone is strong enough to benefit from cancer treatment.

Looking over guidelines on Web sites can give you a general idea of treatment options, but they don't provide the clinical wisdom gained from many long days working in an oncology office. Over the last fifteen years, I have realized that it is not enough to merely know standard treatment guidelines. More important is to understand how to personalize them, and experience is a great teacher. It is experience talking when I suggest to a patient that she might be a better candidate for a mastectomy because of the size of her breasts, because of her asthma, or because the cancer is in her left breast and radiation could worsen underlying heart disease. Women with especially large breasts may need special attention during radiation treatments to keep the doses correct. Women with very small breasts often have poor cosmetic results when a cancer of substantial size is removed followed by radiation treatments.

The following list of cancers and their common problems and pitfalls is not meant to be exhaustive. It includes common cancers and clinical issues, which, hopefully, will enable better decision-making by the patient. However, advice and recommendations from an oncologist are paramount, as he or she is the person who most fully understands each case. The cancers discussed are brain, breast, colon and rectal, metastatic colon, head and neck, lung, small cell lung, melanoma, ovarian, pancreatic, and prostate.

BRAIN TUMORS

These are rare but devastating cancers. Only a limited amount of brain can be safely removed without substantial deficits in function. Complete removal of brain tumors is unusual in many cases, but it is the best treatment. Still, it may also be difficult for the neurosurgeon to know if the resection is complete because the pathology report from a brain tumor removal isn't able to assess whether the margins (or edges) are adequate and free of cancer in the way that such a report can assess a breast cancer specimen. This is because of the nature of brain tissue. It is not a solid, as are other organs in your body.

Many brain tumor patients develop seizures either before or after the surgery and need antiseizure drugs to treat them. At times, some of the older drugs in this category, such as phenytoin, may affect the metabolism of certain chemotherapy drugs. This could result in receiving less than full doses of chemotherapy. Bleeding or infection in an area of the brain weakened by tumor and radiation therapy are rare but dreaded complications. Brain tumor patients also may suffer generalized debility and weakness. Possibly for this reason, blood clots in the legs are common in brain tumor patients.

For the past thirty years little advancement has been made in the medical treatment of aggressive brain tumors. One of the chief reasons is that older classical chemotherapy drugs don't easily move past the body's natural barrier and get into the brain tissue. Newer biological therapies aimed at affecting the blood supply around the tumor are exciting and promising developments. Investigations are ongoing into some of these drugs that are able to penetrate the barrier and block new blood vessels from forming. How these new drugs can best be used for brain tumor patients is still under investigation.

Brain tumors are challenging to treat with chemotherapy because of the blood brain barrier. Many drugs are unable to pass into the brain because of a natural barrier that your body has. This barrier prevents many chemicals and compounds from affecting brain function. Many cancer drugs are complex larger chemicals that don't penetrate the brain. Smaller compounds, like alcohol, for example, easily do. Under normal conditions, this barrier helps protect the brain, but it works against a patient if the goal is to direct chemotherapy drugs to the brain tumor. Temozolomide and Temodar are oral chemotherapy drugs commonly used to treat brain tumors.

Brain tumor patients can have substantial and challenging disabilities in daily function depending on the extent of surgery. Physical, occupational, and speech therapy may be needed. Radiation treatments are routinely used for many brain tumors. Short-term side effects of this radiation include hair loss, scalp redness and itching, and weakness. An easily overlooked side effect of brain radiation is pesky ear wax. The radiation treatments change its composition, making it thicker. Over time, patients or their families may notice hearing loss. Simply having the clinic wash out ears with salt water helps. Long-term side effects are balance and memory loss; they may become profound over the years. These long-term side issues may worsen with time. By lowering the daily dose of radiation, such side effects may be delayed and limited. This may result in the brain radiation taking more weeks to complete. Problems with walking are common in brain tumor patients. This group has a particular need for help with safe transportation and bathing.

BREAST CANCER

In contrast to the ordinary lung cancer patient, most patients with breast cancer show up with an early stage of the disease. This is because of the routine use of mammograms and a better general awareness of the need for early detection. There are, for example, far more breast cancer survivors than those with lung cancer. In general, too, rates of breast cancer survival are higher than the average patient expects. The public health awareness surrounding breast cancer is paying off. This leads, however, to an unusual situation in which the diagnosis of breast cancer is associated with a particularly high degree of anxiety. Knowing many friends and neighbors with the same disease, many of whom survive and some of whom unfortunately don't, leads to the fear.

Not only is early detection common, but good therapies are available for both regional breast cancer and the metastatic breast cancer that has or could spread to other regions of the body. Biological, chemotherapy, and radiation treatments are examples of effective therapies that can cure a portion of regionally advanced breast cancer. Still, certain breast cancer patients do have a much higher risk of doing poorly.

Breast cancers are not all alike. Some respond to estrogen or progesterone hormone-type drugs, while others don't. Some respond to medications that block certain chemicals known as HER-2 growth factors found on the surface of the cancer cells, while others do not. Breast cancers that respond to hormone or HER-2 type drugs are more treatable. The most challenging breast cancers to treat are those that don't respond to hormones or HER-2. These are known as "triple negative." Although many of these are cured each year, there are some hormone and Her-2 positive breast cancers that don't respond. In general, however, the triple negative cancers are most worrisome. If your breast cancer is triple negative, your oncologist will likely recommend more aggressive treatments.

In contrast to other cancers, for which chemotherapy is given to treat an advanced cancer, in breast cancer, chemotherapy is usually used in an adjuvant fashion. Adjuvant chemotherapy is similar to an insurance policy. This means that the chemotherapy is given when no metastatic cancer can be seen. It is given after surgery in an attempt to reduce the chance of the cancer spreading by killing off any microscopic cancer cells that might remain. Whether or not chemotherapy drugs are recommended and how long they might be given depends on the size and features of your cancer. In general, larger breast cancers and breast cancers that spread to the lymph nodes have a higher chance of metastasis or later spread to other of your body's organs. These patients are offered more aggressive treatments of adjuvant chemotherapy. It is easy to see why women who have breast cancers that are at high risk to return are offered more aggressive adjuvant or "insurance policy" type chemotherapy.

At times, one of the most challenging decisions comes when a patient has a small breast cancer with good prognostic factors, such as no lymph node spread and favorable estrogen and Her-2 receptor status. In this situation, the advantages of a course of chemotherapy are relatively small, so it may be difficult to decide whether it is worth taking. For stage 1, estrogen receptor positive breast cancer patients in this predicament, DNA gene tests are now available that can be performed on the breast cancer specimen. This test, known as Oncotype DX, is performed on the pathology specimen and helps to assign these early stage breast cancers to low, medium, and high-risk stage 1 cancer. This might help decide whether to consider chemotherapy. As better DNA techniques are developed, it will become even easier for an oncologist to judge if patients are at a particularly high risk of developing metastatic cancer. In general, the adjuvant chemotherapy is far better tolerated than might be expected. Many times it is worth the added peace of mind for a woman to know that she has done all she could to lower her risk of having metastasis develop.

Surgery for breast cancer can include removal of the breast, called a mastectomy, or removal of only the lump, known as a lumpectomy. A woman's survival chances are similar whether or not she has a mastectomy to remove the entire breast cancer or a lumpectomy to keep the breast intact. Many women are surprised to discover that removing the entire breast doesn't improve their chances of surviving the breast cancer when compared to having only a lump removed.

For almost all breast cancers, a lumpectomy requires a woman to have radiation therapy to the remaining breast in order to reduce the chance of breast cancer returning in the affected breast. Most women tolerate this radiation therapy well and welcome the option of keeping their breast. Some women, however, may be poor candidates for this treatment. Women with advanced emphysema, for example, could be considered marginal candidates for radiation therapy. Along with the breast, sometimes a small amount of normal lung tissue is exposed to radiation. This can result in irreversible lung scarring and difficulties in recovering from lung infections.

The lung fibrosis that can occur isn't usually life threatening, but it can be serious and can result in significant disability. Women with asthma or emphysema may need to be careful when considering breast radiation treatments. In addition, radiation therapy is usually not offered to people with certain rheumatologic conditions, such as lupus or scleroderma, as the skin effects often results in severe skin reactions. Radiation therapy to the left breast can also be a cause for concern. Depending on how much of the heart is treated with radiation, the radiation treatments may offer a higher than normal risk for developing heart disease.

Gene studies to detect whether or not you are carrying a gene that increases the chance of developing another breast cancer can be performed. These are done through blood tests that may detect two different types of genes. If you're a carrier of one of them, your surgeon might offer to remove both breasts. This is to reduce the chance of developing another breast cancer. Some patients who are carriers may also have surgery to remove their breasts even without having a diagnosis of cancer. Myriad is one company offering this test. It's called BRACAnalysis.

Many reconstruction options exist for women who have lost all or part of a breast from cancer. The best cosmetic results are seen in women who have not had radiation therapy. However, certain types of reconstructive procedures (such as the trans flap, a procedure whereby a flap of skin is moved from the abdominal area) present the least number of problems. Wounds heal much slower in areas exposed to radiation. This holds true even if the area involved was treated with radiation therapy many years ago. At times, radiation is needed even if the entire breast is removed. In these cases, reconstruction efforts need to be carefully planned by the radiation therapist to avoid wound healing problems.

Women who are diagnosed with large breast cancers that are too big to remove initially can often have the tumors shrunk first with chemotherapy. They are then removed when they are smaller. It's known as neoadjuvant chemotherapy. In this situation, the chemotherapy is serving two purposes:

reducing the chance of distant spread of the cancer and shrinking the tumor, allowing the surgeon to completely remove it when it is smaller.

Julie: Chemo Worked to Save Her Breast

Julie was a 58-year-old woman with a large mass at the top of her right breast. She had been tardy in coming to the doctor because of family and insurance concerns. Her breast cancer was initially a sizable mass, about the size of a small hen's egg. After being diagnosed, she was disappointed that the tumor had grown to a size too big to be removed in surgery. Any operation that was initially attempted would have resulted in obvious breast cancer left behind. Her insurance issues were settled, and treatment was begun with a combination of oral hormone derived breast cancer drugs and intravenous chemotherapy. Several months of chemotherapy demonstrated that the tumor was shrinking. At the time of her surgery, she was pleased learn that she would be able to have the entire tumor removed and keep her breast. Even though the pathology report found no remaining active breast cancer in the specimen, she understood the need for further radiation, hormone, and chemotherapy treatments. Several years later she is still doing well on the hormone pills.

Women with metastatic breast cancer often have a prognosis far different than they or their friends would expect. Many believe that when the cancer has moved into the bones, their outlook is very poor. It is not unusual, however, for women with metastatic breast cancer to survive for years after finding out about the spread. Often, the biggest problems are the bone injuries and fractures that occur before treatment begins. Good medications, such as Zometa (zolidronic acid), exist to improve the bone strength and reduce the chance of further bone destruction. These bone-strengthening drugs belong to a class of drugs known as bisphosphonates. Careful attention to dental care is needed when using these medicines.

Some women with metastatic breast cancer can survive more than ten years. This type of slower growing cancer often involves the bones, the skin of the chest, and possibly the fluid around the lungs. Usually some form of treatment is given, although simple hormone pills may suffice for a long while.

Julieanne: Good Health, Thick Skin

Julieanne was a 58-year-old real estate agent in a small town. She had little income and always lived with her mom. Despite smoking most of her life, she enjoyed overall good health. When she gradually developed shortness of breath and a red rash on her chest and back, she wasn't sure what to make of it. It didn't really bother her, but she found herself unable to sleep in bed anymore; she needed to sit up in a chair. When she eventually found her way to a physician, her entire chest, breasts, sides, and back were covered with a thick red rash. Her chest X-ray found large fluid collections at the bases of both lungs; her right breast was thicker and had skin like an orange. She was told she had an advanced case of inflammatory breast cancer. Since beginning on chemotherapy her fluid and rash have improved, and she can breathe easier now.

It is not unusual for women, as well as physicians, to not recognize the rash that can occur with breast cancer. Sometimes it is mistaken for a skin infection known as cellulitis. The rash of breast cancer is usually thicker, however.

More aggressive versions of metastatic breast cancer exist and may spread and cause problems much quicker, sometimes in months. Usually, younger women have a far more aggressive course of treatment for it, but not always. Breast cancer can spread to the skin, the spine, the bones, the lung, the liver, and the brain. One particularly difficult place to diagnose metastatic breast cancer is when it involves the fluid surrounding the brain. Liver and lung spread of breast cancer usually is associated with a more aggressive type of breast cancer. Because metastatic breast cancer can cause bone erosion and other organ problems, it is best to be followed closely no matter the therapy the oncologist considers. Many effective drugs exist to help treat the cancer. Available lists called compendia can give an exhaustive list of commonly used drugs to be used, but your oncologist can list for you his specific preferences. Arimidex (anastrozole),

Avastin (bevacizumab), Xeloda (capecitabine), Taxotere (docetaxel) doxorubicin, Ellence (epirubicin), Aromasin (exemestane), florouracil, Faslodex (fulvestrant), Gemzar (gemcitibine), Zoladex (goserelin), Ixempra (ixabepilone), Tykerb (lapatinib), Femara (letrozole), megestrol, paclitaxel, Abraxane (paclitaxel albumin bound), Fareston (toremifene), and Herceptin (trastuzumab) are some of the drugs used.

Medications specifically used to prevent bone destruction in patients whose cancer has already spread to bones exist and are helpful. These bone strengthening drugs belong to a class known as bisphosphonates. (Just so you're not confused, these drugs help to keep bones from breaking in a woman already diagnosed with metastatic breast cancer. This is a different situation than normal women taking medication such as Evista (raloxifene), which helps to reduce the risk of developing breast cancer and to treat and prevent osteoporosis in older women.)

Jennifer: Living with Metastatic Cancer

Jennifer was a 35-year-old woman when we met her. She had developed a breast mass, which unfortunately she ignored because of a tragedy in her family. During the six months it was left untreated, it substantially grew. When she eventually came to treatment, she received chemotherapy, surgery, hormone therapy, and radiation therapy, all in attempt to prevent her cancer from spreading. After her treatments stopped, she stayed in remission for almost four years, but then the cancer spread to her spine. While she was initially devastated by the news, she accepted her treatments bravely. We found a combination of therapies that she found tolerable and that were remarkably effective. The bone pain in her spine went away as treatment continued. Four years later she is still pain free, continues to tolerate her treatments well, has not been in the hospital since, and is enjoying watching her son grow.

Many women who have metastatic breast cancer find that the procedures can be tolerable and that life is fairly normal. If you experience excessive symptoms, such as pain or weight loss from cancer, tell the oncologist. He also needs to know if you are experiencing weakness, nausea, vomiting, or numbness from treatment.

COLON AND RECTAL CANCER

Colon and rectal cancer develop in the large intestine. The early symptoms are weakness, anemia, and bowel obstructions. Later, when the colon cancer spreads to the liver, pain in the right side of the abdomen can develop. Colon cancer can and should be detected early in most people.

A simple test called a colonoscopy can find and allow immediate removal of the polyps that eventually develop into colon cancers. These tests are strongly recommended as they help detect the cancer at early, more curable stages. People who should have a colonoscopy are those who have symptoms, those who have a strong family history of such cancers, or anyone over the age of fifty. Also consider one if a physician recommends the procedure or if there is a change of bowel habits. Some patients notice a change in the shape of their stools. They might be flatter or skinnier-or they might have blood on them. No one should avoid having a colonoscopy because they feel shy or embarrassed or because they worry about drinking the preparatory medication. Colon cancers develop even in those who have good excuses to avoid the test. Most people can tolerate both the preparation and testing needed to complete a colonoscopy. I have seen many patients at an advanced age have the colonoscopy, who have cancers or polyps found. Some patients, particularly those who have had recent heart treatments that require blood thinners, will need special precautions before undergoing the test. Few people are unable to have it done at all.

Bill: Avoided the Test but Not the Cancer

Bill was frequently seen visiting his family members who were my patients long before he was. Occasionally the topic of his health would come up when he was visiting his family in the office. When asked about having a colonoscopy, he gave a manly, funny answer, and shrugged it off. At the age of 55, he was seen as a new patient in the office. He was diagnosed with a low rectal cancer. Chemotherapy and radiation treatments had been recommended by his surgeon to help make Bill's large rectal cancer amenable to an operation. He knew that a very simple polyp removal years before would have kept him from developing a rectal cancer. Instead, Bill was facing extensive treatments along with the very real chance that he might need a permanent colostomy (a bag on the abdominal wall to collect stool from the colon).

While Bill's story is unfortunate and scary, it is meant to teach that the minor inconvenience of the colonoscopy is well worth preventing major problems down the road. Do the test.

Even though most people have access to colonoscopies, many still avoid them and come to the surgeon's or oncologist's office with advanced stage colon cancers. Colon cancer develops from a polyp in the intestine. Left without treatment, they will usually spread through the intestinal wall, then to lymph nodes, then to the liver and, possibly, to the lungs. Colon cancers on the left side of the abdomen often cause intestinal blockage. This is because the stool stream is naturally more solid as it nears the end of the intestine. Colon cancers on the right side of the abdomen, however, will continue to grow. As they bleed, they will cause anemia. Here, on the right side of the abdomen, the stool stream is more liquid and usually the tumors don't cause obstruction. The bleeding caused by colon cancer is intermittent and can be hard to detect. You may notice only a slight darkening of the stool, or no change at all. People with poor eyesight often can't see any change in the stool. At rare times, colon cancer may spread to the lining on the outside of the intestine and cause fluid called ascites to build up.

Rectal cancers, which develop in the last section of the large intestine, often are detected when they cause bright red blood to be seen in the stool. Other times, they may cause bowel blockages. They may also be associated with quite a bit of pain and discomfort. People often initially blame the bleeding and pain on hemorrhoids, sometimes for months, before seeing a physician. Never assume that you know why you have rectal bleeding. Always mention it to a physician. There may be several reasons for the blood.

It is not usual for colon or rectal cancers to be detected after the cancer has spread to the liver or lungs. The reason why colon cancer often spreads to the liver is because the normal blood supply that leaves the colon makes an initial stop there before returning to the heart.

It is not unusual for people to develop more than one colon polyp or cancer at the same time or at different times. It is also not hard for a small polyp or tumor to be missed on a colonoscopy. The procedure is not considered complete until the entire colon has been examined.

There are blood tests to check for colon cancer genes. These tests may be done if you have a strong family history of colon cancer. You may be offered closer follow up and other options if you are positive for the gene. The names of these gene tests are called COLARIS AP and COLARIS offered through Myriad.

Jerry: A Second Colonoscopy Changed the Outcome

Jerry is a 70-year-old man who had developed a rash that caused terrible itching for several years. He had seen many physicians and finally received relief when he was maintained on prednisone pills. Later, when he developed rectal bleeding, a colonoscopy was attempted which detected a large rectal cancer. His surgery and recovery were delayed for several months because of slow wound healing. Months later, as it was time to start chemotherapy treatments to prevent his cancer from returning, it was suggested that he have another colonoscopy—this time a complete examination that went past the initial blockage. His initial test was incomplete; the tumor had obstructed any viewing past it. He was very disappointed to find out that another second colon cancer was detected, this time on the right side of the colon. Again, he had an operation to remove this colon cancer. This called for protracted hospitalization and convalescence. Only then did the itching stop. The second cancer appeared to be responsible for it. He was then able to begin chemotherapy to reduce the chances of both of his colon cancers returning.

He has done well, enjoys playing music in the community, and is very appreciative that a second attempt to complete the colonoscopy was done.

Most colon cancers are found at a time where removal is the initial step in the treatment. This eradicates all visible cancer and evaluates the abdomen for further spread. Prior to surgery, staging tests, such as CAT scans and laboratory tests, may be done to complete the evaluation. Many colon cancer patients are low in iron. Replacing it may help recovery. After several weeks of convalescence, a patient should have a consultation with an oncologist to determine if the risk of colon cancer is high enough to justify a series of chemotherapy treatments with 5-Fu and Eloxatin (oxalipatinum). These should be given with the intention of eradicating any potential remaining colon cancer cells. Usually they are given for three days every other week for about six months. Most people are able to tolerate them and work during this time. Frequent side effects are diarrhea, weakness, and numbness of the hands and feet. Routine surveillance for recurrence is done with regular lab tests, CAT scans, examinations, and colonoscopies.

Rick: Declining Treatment Led to Cancer Spread

Rick was a 66-year-old plumbing supply salesman who also farmed on the side. He was found to have colon cancer that had spread to the lymph nodes. Rick recovered quickly from the operation and was eager to return to work. After the hospitalization for the surgery, he was evaluated by an oncologist to be considered for adjuvant chemotherapy. He was aware that he was at a high risk for return of the colon cancer and was offered treatment on a clinical trial during which all patients would receive close observation. Two thirds would receive adjuvant chemotherapy of slightly different types. (Adjuvant chemotherapy is additional chemotherapy—and insurance policy given to help the chances that surgery has already cured the patient). Rick declined the options offered to him, choosing to not be treated. He believed that because he felt well after the surgery, he couldn't have any more cancer left in him. Feeling poorly when he was initially diagnosed, Rick now felt better. All of his life, he believed, he had been able to tell if something was wrong with his body. When he had an injured ankle, he could tell if it had repaired itself. When he had bronchitis, he could tell if it had improved. He also declined the option of close follow-up with an physician. Several years later, he eventually went back to a physician and complained that his side hurt, ". . . where this hard lump is. What is this lump, Doc?" He had developed widespread metastatic colon cancer. His entire liver was replaced with spots of colon cancer too numerous to count. He had lost twenty-five pounds. Of course, Rick was not a candidate for removal of his multiple liver metastasis. Such surgery is considered when there are only a few stable lesions. He was also too weak to be able to respond to chemotherapy for long.

Rick was offered and declined treatment and follow-up tests because of the commonly held myth that he could "feel" when he had cancer. Only very late into his course, when it was too late to be treated, could Rick "feel" the cancer effects on the body. The tests and evaluations that your physicians suggest are important to help find any signs of trouble early.

Extensive colon cancer found at the initial testing can affect treatment options. This occurs when the patient has colon cancer both in the colon and in areas of spread, such as the liver. Depending on whether a patient is suffering from bowel obstruction or bleeding, a judgment call about surgery may need to be made. Certainly in many situations an urgent operation may need to be done to relieve the bleeding or obstructed bowel. At other times, if the local bleeding or obstruction is severe, but not imminently life threatening, then systemic therapy with chemotherapy may be able to treat both indications. There are downsides to an immediate operation for a patient with advanced colon cancer. In most circumstances, surgical recovery won't permit chemotherapy treatments to be initiated for several weeks because of the low blood counts that develop after chemotherapy (and the effects that it can have on wound healing). When recovering from an operation, the remainder of the colon cancer elsewhere in the body will grow. This delay may further weaken the patient. If an immediate operation is chosen, a large amount of the cancer remains untreated. Because of this, he or she may not ever recover enough strength to benefit from chemotherapy treatments.

Warren: Surgery or Chemotherapy?

Warren, a 64-year-old dentist, was close to retirement. Despite being a medical professional all his life, he had avoided having colonoscopies. (A colonoscopy is a telescopic examination of the colon.)

When he began bleeding, he ignored it. It was only after he had lost 20 or 30 pounds, that his family took notice and demanded an evaluation. When it became apparent that he had not only developed colon cancer in his bowel, but that it had also spread to his liver, a decision needed to be made. Should the primary tumor in the large intestine be removed at surgery? Or should chemotherapy be started that would treat both the colon cancer in the bowel as well as the colon cancer in the liver? He was started on chemotherapy immediately. His blood counts gradually improved as the cancer shrunk with each treatment. The liver masses of colon cancer also responded. At a later time, Warren could be a candidate to have both the colon cancer in the colon, as well the several lesions in the liver, removed at surgery.

Warren had stage IV metastatic colon cancer and needed therapy that would treat all of it. If he had developed a critical problem at the site of the primary colon cancer in the colon, surgery would have been considered. He has done well because all areas of the cancer were treated.

METASTATIC COLON CANCER

Metastatic colon cancer is usually found in the liver, lymph nodes, or lungs. Routine therapy is to consider chemotherapy treatments to relieve the symptoms being caused by the cancer. These symptoms may include weight loss, weakness, pain, and shortness of breath. Spread to the liver and lung is common. Several types of chemotherapy regimens are used. These include combinations of drugs such as those listed below. At times only a single area of spread can be discovered. When the areas of colon cancer spread to the liver or lungs have responded to chemotherapy, the CAT scan will show them to be decreasing in size and number. If there are only a handful of these lesions, it is tempting to consider having them removed at surgery. Under certain conditions this may be considered helpful.

Bevacizimab is a biologic drug that is sometimes used in advanced colon cancer patients. While it has been found to be helpful in many, it may cause complications with wound healing when it has been given soon before surgery. Careful monitoring is needed if this is chosen. Xeloda (Capecitabine), Erbitux (cetuximab) fluorouracil, Camptosar (irinotecan), Eloxatin (oxaliplatin), Vectibix (panitumumab) are all examples of drugs approved to treat advanced colorectal cancer.

Often surgical removal of one or a few areas of spread is considered appropriate if the cancer has been found spread to only a small number of lesions that he surgeon can remove. While it is recognized that many smaller islands of colon cancer could have spread to the liver or lungs, it has also been found that some patients have only these first few tumors. Thus, removal of these areas might cure the patient. Excision of the metastasis is appropriate in only certain circumstances. A patient may need to have a small number of advanced lesions that are amenable to surgery.

In certain areas of the liver, surgery is technically challenging. In addition, the surgeon will assess if the patient will be left with a functional amount of normal liver for survival. Either before or after surgery on the areas of spread of the cancer, a patient may receive chemotherapy treatments to improve the chances that other smaller lesions won't reappear. It is usually a good option not to consider surgery as soon as the spread to the liver or lung is found. By starting chemotherapy first, treatment is being given to the areas of known spread as well as to the microscopic areas of potential spread. Further, by waiting three to six months, the physicians will be able to ensure the stability of the number of lesions. It is disappointing for patients to spend a month recovering from such major surgery only to find that they have suddenly developed many new areas of metastatic colon cancer spread.

Jeff: Chemotherapy and Then Surgery

Jeff, a 66-year-old carpenter, had undergone surgery and chemotherapy for colon cancer. Three years later, during his routine follow-up visits, a sizable mass had been found to have developed in the left side of the liver. The right side was spared, as were his lungs. Careful testing was completed, which found Jeff to have no other evidence of cancer, not even in the remaining bowel. After four months of treatment, the liver mass had shrunk slightly but was still sizable. More significantly, however, no new areas of cancer were found. He was considered for surgery to remove the colon cancer in the liver. While it would be a major operation, he was thought healthy enough for surgery and complete removal of the two inch liver mass. It was performed with the removal of a tumor that was about two inches in diameter. No other areas of cancer were found. Further chemotherapy was given for a time, followed by close observation. It is now ten years later, and Jeff has not developed any further evidence of colon cancer. He is enjoying his retirement.

RECTAL CANCER

Rectal cancer is a special type of bowel cancer. Because of its location, it has a high chance of spread to the local area surrounding the rectum. For this reason, many patients receive radiation therapy in addition to chemotherapy and surgery. The order in which these three types of treatment are given can vary with a surgeon's and oncologist's recommendations. In the past, initial surgery to remove the rectal cancer left many patients with a permanent colostomy bag. (A colostomy bag is a device whereby the stream of stool is collected in a pouch attached to the skin of the abdomen. Newer treatments are able to spare the anus, leaving the patient without the need for a colostomy.)

Surgical treatment for rectal cancers needs to be carefully coordinated with the medical and radiation oncologist. The medical oncologist is responsible for the chemotherapy and medical care, while the radiation oncologist plans and delivers radiation treatments. This team of physicians needs to be able to work together. Recently, instead of removing the rectal cancer at surgery initially, the tumor is treated with chemotherapy and radiation before an operation is attempted. Further follow up chemotherapy treatments are usually done as well. These reduce the chance of spread of the rectal cancer to distant organs such as the liver. Today, fewer patients need the more radical operation that removes the rectum and anus. This improves quality of life tremendously.

Long-term effects from rectal surgery include the sense of needing to urgently move the bowel after a meal. This effect can be disabling for some and lead them to need to go to the bathroom numerous times a day. Common side effects from chemotherapy include dry skin, numb hands, weakness, and anemia, but these are minor compared to the bowel urgency issues. Adaptations that can help include diet changes as well as carefully planned meals and activities.

HEAD AND NECK CANCERS

Smokers and drinkers are common candidates for throat cancers. Rarely are they diagnosed early, as it is common that throat cancer patients choose to have little or no routine health care. Often they are also challenged by limited amounts of family or social support because of their past unsociable behaviors. Others develop the disease with little or none of the above exposures for no apparent reason. Throat cancers spread to local lymph nodes and to the nearby neck region. Rarely do they spread to the lungs, liver, or the remainder of the body.

The best results are seen when these tumors are treated with a combined modality approach with an experienced team. A patient's medical team should consist of a medical oncologist, giving appropriate chemotherapy, a radiation therapist, and a surgeon. After diagnosis and staging is completed, the patient should have a face-to-face consultation with each of these specialists. It is important that a decision not only be made about best treatment options, but also that there is an understanding of the potentially serious consequences of each type of treatment. Surgery may result in serious cosmetic and functional deficits that may affect speech, swallowing, and mobility. Radiation can also affect swallowing and could make the neck stiff. Chemotherapy may affect kidneys; it may also cause nerve damage known as neuropathy and induce nausea and vomiting.

Organ preservation techniques allow the patient to keep their voice box and preserve swallowing and speech. Radical surgery techniques also exist which expert teams of surgeons at major universities might offer after a careful review of each case. Some of these procedures remove quite a bit of tissue, including possibly the voice box or jaw bone. It is wise to carefully consider all other available options—various consultations should be pursued to make an adequate study of nonoperative choices—before finally agreeing to aggressive surgery. Consider getting a consultation with medical oncologists, radiation oncologists, and reconstructive surgeons in addition to a head and neck surgeon. This will help your deliberations. Plans for nutrition and speech therapy should also be discussed before taking that step. Newer biological drugs, such as Erbitux (cetuximab), also hold promise for patients with advanced head and neck cancer.

Aspiration of food and secretions leaking down into the lungs through the trachea or windpipe is a common side effect of both surgery and, especially, of radiation treatments. Frequent pneumonias occur that may be life threatening and also cause lung fibrosis. Speech therapy uses a variety of means to help improve swallowing by restoring a normal gag reflex. Other means to help swallowing are to thicken liquids to pudding consistency through means of dietary supplements. It is often hard for patients to recognize that they are swallowing incorrectly and are actually aspirating. Aspirating contributes to pneumonia when throat secretions or food are sent down the windpipe instead of into the esophagus. A swallowing study can be done in the radiology department which helps to make the diagnosis. By recognizing and treating aspiration, one of the most serious consequences of radiation treatments to the throat can be prevented. Proper therapy by a speech therapist can help to treat this.

Radiation treatments to the neck are some of the most challenging cancer treatments to complete. This is because of the amount of throat irritation that they cause. Therapy usually lasts for six to seven weeks. Although it may seem long, this is the expected duration. At times, chemotherapy and radiation therapy are given simultaneously, as the combination may improve the radiation's effectiveness. Weight loss, neck pain, and a sore throat severe enough to prevent eating are to be expected. A tube, called a gastostomy or G-tube, inserted in the stomach to supplement feedings is common. The extra nutrition available through the tube will allow for quicker recovery from radiation treatments. If one is offered, you should strongly consider it. Many patients receiving this type of therapy can be expected to need a break during the radiation to help heal their sore throats. While it is best to take as few breaks as possible, patients with throat cancer shouldn't push themselves so hard that they become dehydrated, malnourished, or develop an infection. Because of the cancer and treatments, infections are also common at this time. They may show up as a white coating on the throat or just one that is severely inflamed; shaking chills with or without a temperature are also prevalent. Stay in close touch with your oncologist at this point.

Erbitux (cetuximab) and Taxotere (docetaxel) are the names of two chemotherapy drugs commonly used to treat advanced stage head and neck cancers.

LUNG CANCER

Because screening tests are not routine even among high-risk people, lung cancer isn't found early in the majority of patients in which it is diagnosed. Routine screening is recommended only when it is proven that such tests would improve survival chances. So far, studies have not found chest X-rays or chest CAT scans to be helpful enough to be routinely recommended. Additionally, people at high risk for lung cancer, including smokers, don't usually seek out medical care that would result in an early diagnosis. In contrast, it is the smoker who often avoids routine health care. CAT scans for screening purposes are not typically paid for by insurers. Those fortunate high-risk patients who have wise primary care providers who aggressively evaluate chest symptoms seem to have a better prognosis when their lung cancers are found earlier. A patient whose physician considers that the smoker's pneumonia or coughing up of blood might be the result of lung cancer often receives a careful evaluation and follow-up. A certain number of these closely followed patients will quit smoking and realize the importance of monitoring their health. If the chest symptoms of cough, pain, or bleeding are assumed to be from benign conditions, such as smoker's hack, this may result in a delayed diagnosis and patients whose disease is advanced when they are eventually treated.

Symptoms that are frequent at the time of diagnosis are hoarseness, fatigue, cough (which may produce blood), and pneumonia that doesn't go away. Other common symptoms are weight loss and back or side pain. Most, although not all lung cancer patients, are or have been smokers. Rare is the lung cancer patient who hasn't been, or lived with, a smoker. Exposure to asbestos, radiation, radon or other carcinogens, such as certain industrial chemicals, may also contribute to a greater risk. Also, many lung cancer patients have a strong family history of lung and other cancers.

Treatment of lung cancer depends on its stage at the time of diagnosis. It is not unusual for patients to have been somewhere in the medical system for months with vague complaints that may have been attributed to emphysema, pneumonia, asthma, or other diseases. The patient is also frequently dealing with other medical issues related to smoking, such as heart disease, lung disease, renal failure, and vascular disease. Strokes and heart attacks may occur frequently in these patients, as the cancer itself may change the blood composition, thereby increasing the risk of stroke and heart attack.

Lung cancers are most often not diagnosed early. Frequently, however, physicians, patients, and families want to believe that the lung cancer has been diagnosed in an early stage. Enlarged adrenal glands, abnormal areas in lymph nodes, and symptoms of low back pain are ignored. When this happens, local treatment, such as radiation therapy or surgery, is directed toward only the local lung cancer in the chest. Without systemic treatment, such as chemotherapy, lung cancer cells in other areas of the body are left untreated.

Sean and Joy: Different Approaches to Advanced Lung Cancer

Sean was a burly 62-year-old man who had been diagnosed with lung cancer after his pneumonia had failed to resolve. At the time of diagnosis, it was assumed by his doctors that his adrenal mass was an unrelated benign mass known as an adenoma. A decision was made to limit his therapy to local surgery and radiation treatments on the lung mass. His physicians believed he had early stage II lung cancer and a good chance of surviving. Systemic chemotherapy was thought unnecessary, as Sean did not have obvious stage IV lung cancer or symptoms. When these treatments were completed, the adrenal mass began to grow. Despite his weight loss and weakness, the adrenal mass was removed and found to be lung cancer. Chemotherapy was then considered, but he soon developed symptoms indicating that the cancer had spread outside the lungs. The first was a broken hip that kept Sean bedridden and delayed the start of chemotherapy. When he finally began chemotherapy, he was essentially bedridden. As a result of his debilitated medical condition, Sean was only able to tolerate limited doses of chemotherapy for a month or two. As his conditioned weakened, he and his family requested hospice care.

Joy was a 56-year-old woman diagnosed with advanced lung cancer. While she was disappointed when she was found to have metastatic lung cancer with an adrenal metastasis, she kept on fighting. Because her cancer was stage IV, her treatment started with intravenous chemotherapy. She was able to drive herself back and forth to most all of her therapy. After four months of treatment, both her lung and adrenal masses had improved. Joy went on to have first the lung and then later the adrenal mass removed. Following the removal, additional chemotherapy was given for six months. After it was finished, her intravenous port was removed, and she has been in remission for several years.

Both patients had stage IV or metastatic lung cancer at the time of diagnosis, as many lung cancer patients unfortunately do. One benefited from knowing that the lung cancer had spread and was definitely stage IV. The other patient, in a vain attempt to be optimistic, was blinded to the true extent of the cancer. It is not always possible to exactly know the true extent of the cancer. PET scans and biopsies can be done, but they are also inexact. A biopsy might show no cancer but be wrong—the physician missed the lesion. A PET scan might not distinguish between cancer and inflammation in a certain area.

These are grey areas where the physicians judgment is important. Both the physicians and the patient hoped that the cancer was detected early. This optimistic assumption, led to the use of only local radiation and surgery. The chemotherapy that could have been initially given to treat both the metastatic cancer and the primary tumor in the lung had to be delayed until the patient became too weak. If a treatment plan assumes that the lung cancer is early, when in fact it is advanced, the risk of being undertreated is very real and may lead to a potentially fatal outcome. But, on the other hand, if the treatment plans assume that the lung cancer is advanced when it is early, the risk is run of being potentially overtreated. This overtreatment may involve having to take chemotherapy, radiation therapy, and surgery with all of their side effects. However, the chance of survival will likely be greater if the treatment assumes that the cancer is at a more advanced stage.

The treatment plan for lung cancer is decided by the physicians caring for you. This does not always include an oncologist. Even if it does, assumptions are often made that limit the physician's ability to know the correct stage of the cancer. Is a bone scan sufficient to ensure that back pain is not from cancer? (It may not be, consider asking about an MRI.) Is it safe to assume that a mass that a CAT scan shows in your adrenal gland is a benign growth? (It is not, ask for a PET scan). Lung cancer, like many other cancers, has a high chance of spreading or metastasizing.

Chemotherapy for lung cancer is far more effective when the patient is functioning better, is strong enough to be up and walking regularly, and is not bedridden. The several months of time around the diagnosis is a very challenging period. Chemicals made by the cancer alter the body in such manner that there is a higher risk of stroke, heart attack, and blood clots in the lungs. If your lung cancer has been found at an advanced stage, starting treatment with chemotherapy allows the opportunity to reverse some of the harmful biological effects of the disease. This will diminish the chance of complications. It also gives the oncologist the opportunity to evaluate heart and lung conditions to see if smoking has caused any lung or heart damage before a major surgery is undertaken.

Taxotere (Docetaxel), Tarceva (erlotinib), Gemzar (gemcitabine), paclitaxel, Alimta (pemetrexed), and vinorelbine are examples of chemotherapy drugs used to treat advanced stage non-small cell lung cancer. Avastin (Bevacizumab) is used to treat a specific type of advanced non-small cell lung cancer known as adenocarcinoma.

Lung cancer surgery is essential and important for the early stages of lung cancer. Prior to the operation, it is expected that there will be preoperative evaluations done by a family physician and possibly by cardiologists or pulmonologists. Proper staging and oncology evaluations are also important as reviewed in the previous sidebar describing Sean and Joy. Newer surgical techniques allow for far more lung to be preserved than in the past. (This allows for far fewer long-term breathing problems than with older techniques.)

Radiation therapy to the chest is often used to help treat lung cancer. Side effects can include esophageal irritation, as well as radiation injury to the lungs, as a result of radiation scarring. Side effects from radiation therapy to the chest may be greater when chemotherapy is given simultaneously, but radiation therapy is more effective in this combination. Long-term radiation effects in these areas can lead to permanent loss of lung and esophagus function. Symptoms include cough, shortness of breath, and difficulty swallowing. A certain number of these side effects can be expected to continue long after the radiation is completed, sometimes for years. You may be particularly sensitive to the lung effects of radiation if lungs have damage from smoking. Infections may have a prolonged course.

SMALL CELL LUNG CANCER

Small cell lung cancer is very serious and challenging to treat. It begins at the center of the chest near an area called the mediastinum and is often easily overlooked by physical examinations and chest X-rays. It may hide behind the breastbone in the center of the chest and not be visible on chest X-rays. Similarly, the symptoms are often attributed to smoking. Along with the enlargement of a central chest mass, patients notice the rapid development of a cough, phlegm sometimes mixed with blood, tremendous shortness of breath, weight loss, and chest pain. Rarely does it occur in people who haven't either been a smoker or extensively exposed to smoke. The onset can be very rapid, and many families and patients become fearful because of the speed with which it grows. Often, people notice minimal shortness of breath one week and in the next month could need ventilator support in the intensive care unit. It is imperative that diagnosis be as early and quick as possible.

Your evaluation for this type of cancer needs to be done quickly. Several methods may be used to diagnose small cell lung cancer. These include a bronchoscopy, a needle biopsy, or an open biopsy. In a bronchoscopy, a small flexible camera is inserted into the lungs while a person is sedated. A biopsy may be done at the same time. A needle biopsy is often unable to be safely performed for small cell lung cancers because they grow in the center of the chest close to large blood vessels. Thus, radiologists are worried that they might inadvertently cause a large vessel to bleed. An open biopsy is where a surgical procedure or an operation is performed to make the diagnosis.

Small cell lung cancer quickly spreads to the liver, spine, adrenal, and brain. Often by searching for areas of spread, an oncologist may find areas outside the lungs that are worrisome for the spread. These areas are easier to sample with a needle biopsy than the chest. The liver and spine are sometimes the easiest and safest areas to biopsy, as they have lower chances of bleeding and infection complications. Diagnosing a small cell lung cancer may take time while the patient's condition is becoming worse. It is important for all to be flexible to allow a quick diagnosis. This may involve phone calls to other consultants or even hospitalization. Each time a sample of tissue is removed at a biopsy, a waiting period begins until the pathologists report is delivered. Special stains, outside consultant reviews, and other tests all may delay the final report and frustrate efforts to begin treatment. CAT scans, PET scans, biopsies, and pathology reports are essential to determining what the treatment will be, but only chemotherapy or radiation will actually treat small cell lung cancer.

Usually physicians try the safest, easiest biopsy possible to limit the chance of harm to the patient's condition, but the yield or chance of getting a diagnosis may be small. If an oncologist suggests a more definitive test, such as a surgical or open biopsy, he or she may be trying to get a more definitive answer more quickly.

One indication of small cell lung cancer is when the symptoms of cough, weight loss, and coughing up blood are accompanied by a tremendous need to drink. This is because a hormone called ADH is produced, which lowers the sodium or salt content in the blood. It can lead to seizures or confusion. The best remedy is to begin to treat the cancer with chemotherapy and quickly reduce the burden of the hormone. Limiting water is another means to help make the sodium normal. If the sodium is either lowered or raised too quickly, problems with confusion and seizures may develop. A few drugs are available to help the sodium level rise, but the best methods are to treat the cancer.

Current smokers who are diagnosed with small cell lung cancer have a very high chance of developing complications as they are being evaluated. These include heart attacks, strokes, and blood clots in the lungs. Such difficulties can further delay attempts to diagnose the underlying cancer. What appears to be pneumonia on a chest X-ray may actually be a small cell lung cancer on a CAT scan. By the time the tumor's presence is realized, the patient may be too weak to go through the necessary tests and treatment. Weakened by the heart attack or blood clot and by the cancer, supportive care may be the only choice. The best way to increase the chances of survival are by quitting smoking, addressing all other medical issues such as underlying heart disease, and notifying the oncologist of all symptoms so a rapid diagnosis can be made.

Trudy: Almost Too Late for Treatment

Trudy, age 67, had been a smoker most of her life. She tolerated emphysema and heart disease but was largely unaware of her tenuous kidney function. She also didn't know that that the tired legs she had after walking a half mile were evidence of clogged arteries. One Thanksgiving she developed what she thought was a bad cold. Despite chest pains, she continued to smoke. After Christmas, she went to her physician's office because she was only able to move about the house with great effort, and the chest pain was almost constant.

One night, the pain forced her to go to the emergency room, where a heart attack was confirmed. Immediate cardiac catheterization, when a cardiologist physician uses intravenous catheters and X-ray devices to examine the arteries of the heart, was able to open up the main arteries that were blocked. Later that same week, a CAT scan was done to follow up on the abnormal chest X-ray . When it confirmed a large central chest mass, a pulmonary consultation and a biopsy were considered. After the weekend, the biopsy was done. Late in the week the outside review by a more specialized pathology team at another facility confirmed small cell lung cancer. By the time the diagnosis was available and oncology was called, Trudy was in intensive care, bedridden, and on support for her breathing. She had lost twenty pounds, wasn't eating, and her sodium was very low. At night, she was confused.

Although Trudy had many strikes against her, she did have one big factor in her favor. In untreated patients, small cell lung cancer will often respond very quickly to chemotherapy. They only take an hour or two to administer over three days and are usually well tolerated. The common side effects are low blood counts. While Trudy's smoking had affected many of her organ systems, it hadn't bothered her blood counts. After many long deliberations, she and her husband agreed to the treatments. Within one week she was out of the intensive care unit and was walking the halls, pain free. She quit smoking, well almost, and went on to survive for another two years.

Between her smoking habit, her denial, and her underlying heart and lung conditions, Trudy had given herself every opportunity not to be able to be treated. Diagnosing and treating her heart attack and cancer almost took too long for her to be able to be offered effective therapy. Despite all of her medical problems, she enjoyed a tremendous will to live that sustained her so that she could enjoy the rest of her life.

Small Cell Lung Cancer Chemotherapy

Chemotherapy for small cell lung cancer can initially have dramatic effects. Masses shrink. Chest pain and cough resolve. Patients are suddenly able to breathe, walk and eat better. The effects that happen in the first several months can be very encouraging. Often, during this time, patients achieve what appears to be an encouraging complete remission. Work schedules resume, and families go about their usual routines. Hycamptin (topotecan) and etoposide are examples of drugs approved to be used in treating small cell lung cancer. After the treatments have helped and the scans have shown a remission, patients can help aid chances in several ways. Quitting smoking at this time would be a great help. It will help improve chances of getting help from further cancer treatment. Quitting will also help to reduce the chances of a new cancer developing if you are cured. Infections also clear quicker if you don't smoke. Another step to consider is to try to exercise and keep weight stable. Later you might need the extra strength and weight. Also you might consider staying in close contact with your oncologist at this time. Mention any changes in pain, breathing, weight loss, or appetite to her. It is important to mention any new changes early.

In some cases, in an all too familiar scene, the CAT scan might show a slightly bigger shadow, or the back pain might worsen, or confusion can occur. Seizure can happen. Some event that represents recurrence starts. The initial chemotherapy has eradicated the sensitive dumb cancer cells. But another group, the smart or resistant ones are now growing. Contrary to the initial good response, the chance of improvement decreases dramatically when small cell lung cancer is treated a second time. Despite further treatments with other chemotherapy agents, the cancer responds slowly, if at all, to the new round. Radiation may be employed to help alleviate a painful bony lesion or to relieve the symptom of brain metastasis.

To date, despite many studies, only a handful of drugs are available to treat recurrent small cell lung cancer. Alone, standard chemotherapy is able to keep the cancer from returning in only certain fortunate patients. Newer biological agents that act through receptors on the surface of the cells and affect the complex cellular machinery have yet to prove useful in helping maintain the good response seen initially. But someday, the study will happen that will make a difference. Because this cancer returns in a large number of cases, try to become involved in a clinical trial.

Chest radiation therapy for small cell lung cancer is done in those patients whose cancers are caught early enough to be limited to the chest. Many small cell lung cancer patients have an extensive stage in which the lung cancer has unfortunately spread far beyond the chest to other organs, such as the liver, the brain, and the spine. For these patients, radiation treatments to the chest are not offered, as it is felt that chemotherapy is most important when treating all of the disease. For those patients whose small cell lung cancer is limited to the chest, radiation therapy is almost always given simultaneously with chemotherapy. Many times, it begins within the first month or so after diagnosis. If cancer has only begun to respond to chemotherapy and if its effects are still noticeable, consider delaying the beginning of radiation for several weeks. There is no magic in starting the radiation earlier, although studies generally support giving it. Because of the lung and esophageal irritation that radiation may cause, it might be easier to delay such treatments until later after the chemotherapy has helped relieve the cancer symptoms. It's better to start it late and to finish it than to not complete the radiation at all. It does improve the chances of surviving small cell lung cancer.

Because so many small cell lung cancer patients eventually see their cancers progress, it is important to consider becoming involved in clinical trials if diagnosed. The clinical trials should be well thought out, preferably local, and not needlessly delay the start of treatment.

MELANOMA

Most skin cancers rarely spread or metastasize to other parts of the body. Melanoma, which usually starts as a darkened mole, can metastasize or spread if left untreated. It can be easily treated with excision if recognized early. When melanoma begins in hard-to-see places, it can be hard to recognize. Some of the common areas where patients miss their lesions include the eye, back, soles of the feet and pelvic region. When diagnosed with melanoma, patients are often surprised by how aggressively a small mole is treated. Extensive surgical procedures with lymph node removal are common. The reason behind this is the tendency of melanoma to spread to a nearby region.

Melanoma is more serious if the lesion is ulcerated, spreads to the nearby lymph node, or grows deep into the skin. Patients who have had such poor risk, locally advanced melanomas removed are candidates for additional treatment known as adjuvant therapy. Many agents have been investigated as potentially useful drugs, but only Intron A (interferon) has been approved so far. Ongoing studies continue to look for other potentially useful agents.

When melanoma spreads, it can be very resistant to treatment. A small number of fortunate patients do, however, respond dramatically to immune-type therapy—Aldesleukin-or Il-2. Because of the substantial side effects, it is administered only by an experienced team in larger centers. These side effects include low blood pressure and cardiac issues that can require monitoring in the intensive care unit.

Because it is often difficult to treat melanoma, patients are frequently offered therapy in a clinical trial setting. While newer agents hold great promise for some melanoma patients, these studies need to be finished. Hopefully any useful drugs will rapidly be made universally available. This cancer is an example where it does make sense to have your oncologist aggressively help look for nearby clinical trials.

Blood tests are also available to see if the patient is carrying a gene that increases risk of developing melanoma. Myriad offers the test named Melaris.

OVARIAN CANCER

As symptoms are vague and easily confused with everyday discomforts, ovarian cancer is rarely found early. Bloating, bowel changes, and weight changes can all easily be confused with other diseases. It would be unusual for someone with these symptoms to first think of ovarian cancer as the reason for their problems. In elderly patients, ovarian cancer can be especially challenging to detect early. Usually, a crisis or near crisis leads to medical attention. Often this is a bowel obstruction or near obstruction. Sometimes, abdominal pain or massive bloating brings women to the doctor's office. Eventually, physical examinations, CAT scans, and lab tests will lead physicians to suspect ovarian cancer. Surgery is the most common way to make a diagnosis, although at times it can also be made from fluid called ascites which is drained from the abdomen.

Women with ovarian cancer will gain weight despite eating less. They notice that they are bloating and retaining fluid, yet they are not hungry. As a result of the ascites, women can have a full feeling in the abdomen that leads to shortness of breath and complaints of feeling full and tired. The cancer can also seep into the undersurface of a lung—this leads to fluid at the base of both lungs. Diuretics or water pills are tried but only help for a short time. High salt diets, such as in soups, restaurant foods, soda pop, or salty snacks will make the ascites worsen quickly.

CAT scans, as well as ultrasounds, commonly underestimate the extent of the ovarian cancer present. Frequently, massive deposits of cancer are lining the abdominal peritoneal cavity, which can only be seen at the time of surgery.

Ovarian cancer usually can't be entirely removed at the time of initial surgery because massive numbers of small-to-medium sized deposits of cancer are often spread throughout the peritoneal cavity. They are too numerous to remove; they may even be on the undersurface of the diaphragm. In addition, complete removal would require taking out too much of the bowels. Removal of the uterus and ovaries—as well as any large deposits of tumor masses in the pelvis—is sometimes all that can be done in what often turns out to be a disappointing partial surgical resection. Nevertheless, "debulking," or removal of only part of the ovarian tumor masses, does help to treat this cancer. In addition to helping to make the diagnosis, it relieves symptoms and decreases the extent of the tumor that needs to be treated by other means, such as chemotherapy. Instead of tens of billion cancer cells, the patient will be left with only one or two billion cancer cells to treat. The surgeon's judgment and experience are important here. Some are more aggressive than others in an attempt to completely remove all of the cancer.

Ovarian cancer can be followed by lab tests, CAT scans, and examinations. Often, it is challenging for chemotherapy to completely remove and eradicate this disease. After chemotherapy treatments are finished, women flollow-up with lab tests and CAT scans are performed. Keep in mind that women are commonly surprised to hear that their cancer can still be present despite years of apparently normal tests.

Fortunately, chemotherapy is highly effective for ovarian cancer. It is usually given by vein either weekly or every three weeks. Carboplatin, Doxil (doxorubicin liposome injection), Gemzar (gemcitabine), pacli-

taxel, and Hycamtin (topotecan) are some of the drugs used to treat ovarian cancer. Ovarian cancer is also one in which chemotherapy can occasionally be placed directly into the peritoneal cavity. This increases the
concentration of chemotherapy to the cancer.

There are two reasons why chemotherapy might be recommended in
ovarian cancer treatment. The first is adjuvant use, which, as with other
cancers, is when chemotherapy is given to help prevent the cancer from
returning. It's an insurance policy. Such adjuvant chemotherapy is sometimes given for several months or more. It should be tolerable for the
patient. Many different schedules and doses are available. Talk to an oncologist about side effects if you are having significant problems. These
may include nerve damage or neuropathy and fatigue. Other side effects
can be low blood counts, hair loss, and nail damage. Routine monitoring is needed as sometimes cancer may give signs of progressing during
treatment.

The second reason for chemotherapy is palliation or relief of symptoms of incurable or metastatic cancer. The duration of treatment depends
on the extent of the cancer and how fast it responds to the therapy. If the
cancer is too extensive for the surgeon to remove, chemotherapy will be
required to relieve symptoms. Some cancers respond more rapidly than
others, although the biggest improvement in symptoms would be in the
first month or two. Some patients may require on ongoing treatment to
keep their ovarian cancers at bay. Others will be able to stop after the
cancer appears to be in remission for a time. While some patients with extensive ovarian therapy achieve long-term remissions and even a cure, this
requires intensive treatments, often for long durations. A little luck is also
needed.

A blood test, offered through Myriad, can tell if you are a carrier for
the ovarian and breast cancer gene known as BRCA 1 and 2. This simple
test called BRACAnalysis, may help you and your family members make
better decisions. Women who are positive for this gene have a much higher
risk of developing both breast and ovarian cancers. Ask your oncologist
more about having this test done if you have ovarian cancer.

It is well known that many women with ovarian cancer show up at an
advanced stage, as the symptoms of ovarian cancer are often confused with
other common ailments. Many times, your medical condition only appears worse after going through a major operation with all of its potential
complications. When you are told that the cancer has not only spread, but

that it is been only partially removed, your spirits also can sink. One strategy is to start your chemotherapy treatments soon after surgery in an attempt to help you recover quicker. On occasion, this remaining cancer can slow recovery from surgery by locking up the bowels. By treating the cancer, you help relieve the obstructing tumors mass.

Lilly: A Goal Achieved

Lilly was a 78-year-old grandma who lived alone. During the Christmas season, she kept repeating to herself that she was determined to have a good holiday. Christmas Eve she found herself in an excruciating amount of pain with a complete bowel obstruction. Eventually, she gave in and sought an evaluation. At the time of her initial surgery, she was so obstructed that nothing more than a biopsy to obtain a diagnosis was able to be safely done. She, her friends, family members, and surgeon all feared for her imminent demise. She was only able to be fed through an IV tube. She couldn't even be fed through a stomach feeding tube. But the determination that had accompanied her denial also accompanied her fight. She was determined to see her granddaughter, a high school freshman, graduate. She was fortunate that her ovarian cancer responded well to chemotherapy. The treatments were tolerable for her, helping to relieve her pain and her obstruction. Her bowels gradually opened up, and she was able to nourish herself orally. She pushed to keep trying and made it to the high school graduation. She especially prided herself on achieving another goal when she saw the same granddaughter graduate from college four years later.

Ovarian cancer can cause bowel obstructions, which is occasionally true for colon and pancreatic cancer as well. At times, either surgery or a procedure known as bowel decompression with a tube inserted in the nose is used. Having a bowel obstruction can be very uncomfortable. If the cancer has stopped responding to chemotherapy and is too extensive for the surgeon to help, other means are used to help relieve the discomfort. The stomach, for example, can be decompressed to alleviate any nausea and vomiting by attaching the suction decompression tube directly to the gastric tube. This avoids a messy tube in the nose. Other means of relieving these obstructing symptoms include using morphine and nausea medications to relieve pain and nausea.

PANCREATIC CANCER

Rarely do patients show up with early stage pancreatic cancer. Only a few patients have been lucky enough to have had symptoms, such as jaundice, developed early from a cancer blocking the bile duct. Most pancreatic cancer patients have months of vague symptoms of pain, weakness, loss of weight, and nausea. It is not unusual for people to attribute these symptoms to benign causes, such as gall bladder, stomach ulcers, or other conditions. Jaundice, or yellow color to the skin, however, is alarming to family and friends and almost always brings a patient to seek medical attention. Depending on the location of the cancer in relationship to the pancreatic duct, some pancreatic cancer patients will develop jaundice early, some late. It just depends on the location of the cancer in relation to the bile duct. Most patients will relay a story about how hard they have been trying to lose weight and about how successful they have been lately. The truth is a chemical made by the tumor is responsible for robbing the appetite and causing weight loss.

The treatment for pancreatic cancer depends on whether it is advanced or not. Trying to assess the chances for surgical success before an operation are challenging. Even with modern technology, it can't always be known with certainty before surgery whether the cancer can be removed. Unfortunately, just as with lung cancer, in most cases, these cancers are too advanced at the time of diagnosis to be removed. A combination of MRI, CAT, and ultrasound tests can help decide if the cancer is removable before an operation is undertaken. If there is any doubt as to whether the pancreatic cancer can be removed, a consultation with a medical oncologist, a radiation oncologist, and a surgeon should be requested. While complete removal of a pancreatic cancer is the best curative option, it is best to operate on a pancreatic cancer only if it hasn't spread, and it is clear that the patient is strong enough to tolerate the surgery. If it has, there are better options. This will only set you back. But, there usually isn't much time before it can develop into a more serious life-threatening condition. Patients often need to decide quickly on starting a treatment. Many have indeterminate masses that might possibly represent cancer spreading in the area near the pancreas, thereby making it hard to determine spread. A combination of radiation therapy and chemotherapy can be a good option for pancreatic cancers that are locally advanced.

If it is unclear whether to pursue surgery for pancreatic cancer, chemotherapy could be initiated during deliberation. It is safer to do something than to remain untreated and let weeks turn into months as one test and consultation after another are completed. This chemotherapy will serve several purposes. It will retard further tumor growth and may help prevent complications, such as weight loss or blood clots that are known as deep vein thromboses (DVT). Patients who have advanced pancreatic cancer found only by undergoing surgery that it had advanced throughout the abdominal cavity. They find it hard to recover adequately enough from an operation to then start the appropriate chemotherapy. On the other hand, some patients, who are not initially surgical candidates, are first treated with chemotherapy. These patients still might be considered for surgery at a later time after their medical condition improves.

The survivors from pancreatic cancer are those who are rapidly treated after cancer is suspected. X-rays, scans tests, and opinions don't treat pancreatic cancer. Radiation therapy and surgery only treat localized pancreatic cancer. Only systemic chemotherapy will effectively attack advanced or metastatic pancreatic cancer. Starting treatment as soon as possible after diagnosis is essential.

This is a common theme among several types of cancers that often are found at an advanced stage deep inside the patient, such as lung and pancreatic cancer. Surgery should be strongly considered only if it is very clear to you and your physicians that it will help. If not, consider other treatments such as chemotherapy or radiation. Surgery can be reconsidered at a later time if the cancer responds well.

Diagnosing pancreatic cancer can be particularly challenging. This is especially true if a patient is not being seen by a physician specializing in this area. Gastroenterologists, medical oncologists, and surgeons all may help. At times, a biopsy to determine if the cancer has spread to the lymph nodes or liver is needed. At other times, an ultrasound guided wire can biopsy a suspicious mass in the intestines through a tube that is passed through the mouth into the stomach. Although an open surgical biopsy is the last choice procedure for a diagnosis, it may be necessary. A blood test known as "CA

19-9," when it is elevated is helpful to confirm the diagnosis. On rare occasions, a combination of the elevated CA 19-9 blood test, weight loss, abdominal pain, and a mass on scans can lead several physicians to concur that a clinical diagnosis of pancreatic cancer is appropriate. This may allow consideration of initiating medical treatment and is especially useful in elderly patients, who may refuse or who may not be candidates for surgery.

Radiation therapy for pancreatic cancer is challenging to tolerate, especially when recently diagnosed. It may be better tolerated after symptoms have been relieved by receiving several months of chemotherapy. It is a good option for local control of a patients' cancer if he or she is not a candidate for surgery for medical or surgical reasons. Long-term effects from this radiation include bowels inflammation, diarrhea and abdominal pain. As with any radiation to the abdomen, small bowel obstructions caused by scar tissue that develops after the radiation treatments can be very difficult to treat.

Chemotherapy for pancreatic cancer has improved over the last ten years, but it is still only modestly effective. Generally, a combination of intravenous and oral agents are used. Treatments can be given regularly until progression of the symptoms or scan findings are seen. The chemotherapy treatments, based on Gemzar (gemcitabine) and Tarceva (erlotinib), can be especially useful to help control symptoms of pain and weight loss caused by the cancer. Smoking appears to both limit how long the treatment is effective and create additional complications.

PROSTATE CANCER

Prostate cancer is a common disease of elderly men. Many times, older prostate cancer patients will have many other medical issues, including heart disease, lung disease, diabetes, and vascular disease. For them, prostate cancer is one of many in a long list of illnesses.

If found in younger men, prostate cancer is more aggressive or likely to spread. They're more likely to have their prostate cancer as their primary medical problem and be in otherwise good health.

In the past, many men have been informed that they didn't need to worry about dying from prostate cancer as it progressed so slowly that something else, such as a heart attack, broken hip, or stroke, would probably take their lives. More recently, however, it has been recognized that untreated prostate cancer may have been contributing to the increased chance of blood clots leading to strokes and heart attacks.

Prostate cancer is most often diagnosed through a screening test performed by a primary care provider. Less often, a man may complain about trouble urinating or notice blood in the urine. In either event, a urologist usually helps to make the diagnosis through an uncomfortable test known as an ultrasound guided transrectal biopsy. In this procedure, a biopsy probe is passed through the rectum and into the prostate—six or eight times. Prostate cancer can also be diagnosed when an area of bone or lymph node is biopsied, usually with a CAT scan guided needle.

Prostate cancer cells are sensitive to the body's hormones. The testosterone made in a man's testicles can help some of the prostate cancer cells grow; these are called hormone sensitive cells. They can be treated by removing the testicles at surgery or with several types of medications. These treatments are collectively known as hormone ablation. Other prostate cancers are able to grow independently of the presence of the testosterone hormone. These cells are known as hormone independent cells.

Prostate cancer can be cured only if it is found early and is limited to the prostate gland and the surrounding region. Both radiation treatments and surgery are means by which it can be cured. Hormone treatments are sometimes given for several years after radiation treatments are completed. Casodex (bicalutamide), Zoladex (goserelin), Vantas (histrelin), Lupron (leuprolide acetate), and Trelstar (triptorelin) are examples of hormone treatments used for advanced prostate cancer.

Radiation, surgery, and hormone treatments can all affect sexual function. Numerous treatments are available that may help with sexual problems, but these are not universally effective. If a patient values sexual function over survival, it is important to clearly discuss this with the urologist and oncologist.

If choosing to irradiate prostate cancer, a patient should first undergo a colonoscopy or examination of the colon. If this is not done, he may eventually discover an undetected and separate colon cancer. It is unfortunate and confusing when a prostate cancer patient finds out that he also needs surgery for an undiscovered colon problem after completing radiation for a nearby prostate cancer. Radiation to the pelvis will make any type of surgery in the area difficult to heal. The scar tissue from the radiation will even make a colonoscopy more technically challenging, uncomfortable, and risky.

Surgery for prostate cancer is generally not considered after the age of approximately 70 to 75, as men recover their urinary control best at younger ages. After age 70 to 75, the chance of permanent incontinence is too high. Most urologists avoid operating on men above this age for that reason.

Royce: Treatments Contributed to Osteoporosis

Royce, age 78, suffered prostate cancer seven years earlier. He tolerated his radiation treatments well enough and had almost forgotten about them. As an additional treatment, he also was given hormone injections for several years. Then, when he developed a pain in the pelvis, his physician worried about cancer and a bone scan was done. Royce's primary care physician was concerned about a possible return of the prostate cancer. The bone scan and CAT scan both demonstrated an abnormal area of bone in the pelvis. The first worry was that his prostate cancer had spread to his nearby bones. When prostate cancer spreads, the PSA blood test should rise. But because the PSA prostate cancer blood test was normal, a biopsy was needed. No prostate cancer was seen. Royce had developed a fracture in the pelvic bone from osteoporosis. His underlying osteoporosis had been worsened by years of hormone treatments combined with radiation damage to the bones. His lack of exercise didn't help his bone health either. After taking calcium and medication for osteoporosis, he stopped developing fractures and gradually the pelvic fracture healed.

Being aware of the chance of osteoporosis related to your cancer treatments is important. Numerous therapies exist to help prevent painful and costly fractures.

Both hormone ablation injections, as well as the radiation treatments, are able to weaken the bones. It is important to be aware of the state of bone health during prostate cancer. Effective treatments for osteoporosis can be given to reduce the chance of bone loss and fracture.

The PSA score is a useful lab blood test which follows your course. At the time of diagnosis, the higher the PSA, the greater the chance that prostate cancer might spread. Various charts are available that take the PSA and another important piece of information, called the Gleason score, into account to give a rough idea of how likely prostate cancer is to return. The Gleason score is a measure of how aggressive an individual's prostate cancer is. A starting PSA higher than 25 indicates approximately a 50/50 chance of the cancer eventually spreading. A PSA higher than 50 is thought to be associated with prostate cancer eventually returning. The PSA should, theoretically, return to zero after surgery or radiation therapy. It should not be in the normal range. Only prostate cells, normal and malignant, can make PSA. If the prostate gland has been removed or irradiated, the PSA should be zero. Any number above this is evidence that there is further prostate cancer.

Patients can also have a normal or zero level of PSA test for years and still be harboring hidden areas of prostate cancer. If the PSA rises after surgery or radiation treatments, it is not unusual for physicians to try to find any further cancer by doing CAT scans or bone scans. Don't be surprised if these tests are normal. Prostate cancer is far more easily detected by the PSA blood test than by X-rays. A patient and oncologist may know that the prostate cancer is still present long before it can be seen on the scans and far before the cancer can be felt. A rapidly rising PSA score is a bad sign. This signals that there is growing prostate cancer somewhere. In the right situation, an oncologist may use this fact alone to offer treatment with chemotherapy.

Buddy: Complications Prevented

Buddy was an 80-year-old man who didn't like doctors. No doctor had ever had good news for him, he reasoned. So he avoided them until he developed diverticulitis, an infection of the lower colon. During the hospital stay, he was in quite a bit of pain and it was noticed that his labs were abnormal. A bone scan and PSA confirmed that it was likely he also had prostate cancer. With a PSA greater than 12,000, which is much higher than the expected normal level of 4, he was treated with only hormone therapy. For another five years he lived without symptoms. His hormone therapy was limited to injections every three months and a daily pill.

Despite its advanced state, Buddy's disease was still amenable to the injections. These medications along with medicines to strengthen the bones prevented complications, such as vertebral compression fractures, which could have resulted in serious disability.

PROSTATE CANCER GRADES: THE GLEASON SCORE

The Gleason scale is a way in which a prostate biopsy is rated. The cancer is graded for its level of aggressiveness. The higher the score, the more aggressive your cancer is behaving. When a biopsy is taken through a needle, only a tiny amount of tissue is removed. The score obtained by this biopsy may not be as accurate as a biopsy that is obtained when the entire prostate gland is removed. If the treatment involves surgical removal, the patient may get an even more accurate picture of the nature of his cancer because the biopsy sample is larger. If treatment involves radiation therapy, the pathology report relies on the initial needle specimen.

Men with especially high Gleason scores of eight to ten are at a much higher risk of having their cancer metastasize. These cases worry oncologists because the chance that the aggressive hormone independent cells will spread is especially high. If a Gleason score of the prostate cancer is high, it would be a good idea to become involved in a clinical trial that is researching adjuvant or additional preventative treatments.

Effective chemotherapy for prostate cancer has only been in use for several years. Because of this, only a limited number of chemotherapy drugs, such as Taxotere (docetaxel), have been found to be effective. Most of these are in men who need treatment to relieve symptoms of advanced prostate cancer. It is a judgment call as to when to start chemotherapy for metastatic prostate cancer. If the treatments are begun late in the course of the disease, the patient may be too weak for them to be of any help. If the treatments are begun early, the side effects may be more substantial than the symptoms of the prostate cancer.

A man at any age who is able to participate in everyday activities might consider starting chemotherapy treatments earlier rather than later. Waiting might weaken the patient. Waiting to treat the prostate cancer also runs the risk of developing other complications that may limit chances of ever receiving treatment. It is much easier to have treatment for cancer when the patient hasn't also suffered a stroke or heart attack. For example, a patient may also have a serious underlying heart disease in addition to the prostate cancer. A cascade of events may develop whereby the slowly worsening prostate cancer precipitates a heart attack or stroke that limits the ability to have either the cancer or heart disease treated. These complications may also limit the enthusiasm of the physicians, family, and patient to treat either problem. Waiting, without treatment, is unlikely to relieve symptoms if the PSA continues to rise. It would be unusual for someone with advanced prostate cancer to gain strength as the prostate cancer worsens.

Over-the-counter natural products are available that may affect the growth of prostate cancer somewhat. It is known that the hormone estrogen may, for a time, limit its growth. Estrogen compounds are available without a prescription. Some of these products, however, may also increase the risk of stroke and heart attacks. Avoid them. I don't favor patients taking such compounds unless their oncologist is aware of them. Even if they disagree that you should be on them, you should at least let your doctors know if you plan to take them.

EMPOWER YOURSELF

These clinical insights should help when discussing your case with your oncologist or surgeon. Knowing this background information about specific cancers should help empower you to ask intelligent questions and to know whether or not to be aggressive with various treatments.

WHAT'S NEXT

In the next chapter, we will discuss leukemias, lymphoma, and myeloma. These diseases are common, but treatments are far better than several years ago. While there are many more survivors than in the past, it helps to know the common pitfalls and challenges.

Chapter 14

Lymphomas, Myeloma, Leukemias, and Other Blood Cancers

Frequently Overlooked Problems

Oncologists divide cancers into two broad categories. The first includes solid tumors such as were covered in the last chapter, a tumor in which a mass or growth can be measured and felt, such as breast, colon, or lung cancers. The second category includes liquid tumors, such as leukemia and myeloma, which often don't involve a mass. Liquid tumors are most often found in the bone marrow or the blood stream. Hematologists, specialist physicians who treat blood clotting disorders, treat these liquid tumors. This chapter focuses on five common blood cancers: myelodysplasia (another term for *preleukemia*), myeloma, chronic lymphocytic leukemia *(CLL)*, chronic myelogenous leukemia *(CML)*, and acute myelogenous leukemia *(AML)*.

LYMPHOMAS

Quite a bit of confusion exists about the term lymphoma, or leukemia. Lymphomas are a series of different diseases of the white blood cells inside lymph nodes. One particular type of chronic leukemia also has a lymphoma component. Try not to get hung up on the terminology. It can be compared to the three forms of water. Regardless of whether water is in the form of ice, steam, or liquid, it is still water. Similarly, regardless of whether the cancer is found in the bloodstream and is called leukemia or found in the lymph nodes, the diseases are called lymphoma.

Lymphomas are divided into many different types, including Hodgkin's and non-Hodgkin's classes. Hodgkin's disease is a malignancy that occurs most commonly in the young, starts in the chest lymph nodes, and follows a characteristic pattern of spread. These types are further divided into subtypes. It is highly curable in many patients, even when it is advanced. Hodgkin's disease was the first example of a cancer where combinations of chemotherapy were developed that were able to cure patients.

In the past, many younger women in their teens and twenties were treated with radiation therapy. One goal of this was to avoid chemotherapy and keep the women fertile. Often this radiation included treatments to the chest and breasts. These resulted in the women being cured of their Hodgkin's. Unfortunately, the radiation therapy increased the women's chances of developing breast cancer.

There are more than ten different subclasses of non-Hodgkin's lymphomas, but for the purposes of treatment there are usually three major types. The first is slow growing and is known as the indolent lymphomas. These initially grow at a very slow rate but often recur. Over time, their unstable DNA can mutate and transform into more aggressive types of lymphomas.

Indolent lymphomas are initially very responsive to even minimal chemotherapy and radiation treatments. Even without any intervention, it is not unusual for a patient to survive up to ten years. It is also common to not even need any treatment with these slow growing lymphomas, although oncologists are becoming more aggressive about treating them. A cure for indolent lymphomas has remained difficult to achieve. Even after remission, these lymphomas eventually return in most patients. Newer treatment strategies employ a combination of intravenous chemotherapy drugs along with monoclonal antibodies. Treanda (bendamustine) is a drug recently approved for the treatment of non-Hodgkin's lymphoma.

Monoclonal antibodies are examples of targeted therapies directed toward the specific chemicals, called receptors, on the surface of lymphoma cells. These antibodies can be either cold and not radioactive or hot and linked to a particle of radiation, but in the majority of cases, cold antibodies are used. No special radiation precautions are needed. These cold antibodies are given in the medical oncology office. One example is a drug named Rituxan (rituximab). These targeted antibodies are key to improving the chances of many lymphoma patients to both get into and stay in remission.

Cold, or nonradioactive, antibodies have several advantages over the hot antibodies. They can easily be given repeatedly without concern about accumulating a total dose of radiation. Repeated doses of these drugs will severely lower the white blood cell counts. This rarely occurs with the cold targeted drug, rituximab. The nonradioactive antibodies also are much less likely to contribute to a radiation-caused leukemia or cancer. Although this is a theoretical risk and may take years to develop, it can occur. Leukemias and other cancers caused by radiation or chemotherapy are expected to be very difficult to treat.

Lymphomas can be indolent diseases, which means they may last from a few years to ten or fifteen years. Over time, the lymphoma cells naturally become more resistant to treatments. This resistance often develops when standard chemotherapy drugs are used. Use of antibodies, such as the drug Rituxan (rituximab), however, allows a long holiday from chemotherapy. This helps the body's bone marrow function to recover and minimizes the exposure to chemotherapy drugs. During the protracted time in which the lymphoma is kept in remission by such antibody drugs, patients generally suffer few, if any, symptoms from either their disease or their treatment. As is the case with many cancer patients, quality of life is better when the disease is inactive. Also, by staying in remission, you avoid the complications and symptoms of the disease of lymphoma itself, as well as the need for retreatment with combination chemotherapy.

When the monoclonal antibodies are linked to radiation particles, several concerns arise. The radiation can affect your body's bone marrow function, thereby limiting your resistance to infections. The radiation exposure may also, over time, induce a higher chance of developing a second leukemia. Zevalin (ibritumomab tiuxetan), and Bexxar (tositumomab and iodine I-131 tositumomab) are examples of two of these drugs.

Jeanne: Treatment Side Effects
Affect Quality of Life

Jeanne was 75 years old when she was diagnosed with lymphoma. Fortunately, her cancer was in an early stage. It appeared to be limited mainly to the neck. Because her disease was in an early stage, it was thought to be curable. Jeanne received a brief course of chemotherapy, which was combined with radiation treatments. She did well for years, and her lymphoma never recurred. She did, however, develop increasing problems with lung infections. Her previous history of smoking had been minor, but when combined with the small amount of radiation damage to her lungs and her age, it created serious problems. Over time, she needed oxygen first only at night, then constantly. She gradually became severely limited by her respiratory status and developed, increasingly, more serious lung infections.

Her lymphoma could have been treated with chemotherapy alone —and probably should have. True, Jeanne might have had a small chance of them developing other limiting side effects, such as heart damage, but by treating her with chemotherapy and monoclonal antibody drugs, such as rituxan, she could have both enjoyed a remission and avoided the lung infections. She also might have had a higher risk of the lymphoma returning.

Lymphoma can cause many symptoms. These include fevers, chills, night sweats, and fatigue. Other symptoms common to the slow growing lymphomas are kidney failure as a result of blockage of the tubes called ureters that drain the urine from the kidney. Less common are blood clots and strokes caused by changes to the blood's likelihood to clot. At times, pain or numbness can be caused by lymphoma pinching off nerves that travel to arms and legs. Lymphomas can also occur in the bowel and cause vague symptoms. These include diarrhea, constipation, or trouble with nutrition. Lymphomas confined to the intestine can be very challenging to diagnose. At times surgeons will try to both diagnose and remove these bowel lymphomas. Limiting the surgery and relying on chemotherapy and monoclonal antibodies for treatment seems to be the better approach.

Newer molecular biological tests that test the receptors on the surface of the cancer cells, known as flow cytometry, can diagnose lymphoma in the intestine using only a small sample obtained during an endoscopy. (An endoscopy is when a small telescope is used to examine the patient's stomach or intestines.)

Lymphomas can also begin outside the lymph nodes in unusual places. These areas include the brain, skin, lung, cervix, and throat. When they begin in the skin, they can appear as long-term nonhealing patches or tumors that are known as T-cell lymphomas. These may grow over several years and are treated with an entirely different group of both chemotherapy and molecularly targeted drugs. Targretin (Bexarotene), Ontak (denileukin diftitox), and Zolinza (vorinostat) are examples of drugs for t-cell lymphomas.

Intermediate grade lymphomas are also common. Fortunately these lymphomas are more curable than the slow growing variety. Because this type of lymphoma is more curable, the treatments are more intense and regimented. Depending on the stage of the lymphoma, either chemotherapy or chemotherapy and radiation will be used. The combinations of drugs employed vary, but usually four or five drugs are given every three weeks for four to six months. Again, monoclonal antibodies directed against receptors on the surface of the lymphoma cells improve survival chances.

Chemotherapy can be especially effective with lymphomas. In this circumstance a complication known as tumor lysis syndrome may occur. This is where so many lymphoma cells are killed off by the treatments that they effect the bodies other organs. The kidneys in particular need to be protected from this effect by hydration and certain medications.

Patients who are suffering from lymphomas develop particular types of complications from the disease and the treatment. In addition to certain infections, other complications often include certain pneumonias because of the compromised immune system from the lymphoma. Antibiotics may be given once or twice a week during treatments to prevent these pneumonias. Other infections that occur commonly are viral, such as cold sores in the mouth or shingles. The chance of contracting shingles can be diminished if the patient has been vaccinated or if he or she is able to take a further medication to prevent it. Shingles shows up as a close group of blisters on a red base on only one side of the body, usually in a band. After the rash and infection, it leaves many patients with the dreaded postherpetic neuralgia or after the shingles pain syndrome. Avoid the pain syndrome by recognizing the rash and starting on the shingles antiviral pain medicine as soon as possible. Yeast infections in the mouth, skin, and genitals also are commonly seen in lymphoma patients. Early treatment helps here also.

Other important complications when treating lymphoma patients include toxicities from certain drugs. One commonly used is vincristine. This drug can cause a paralyzed bowel known as an ileus. The bloating that develops is very uncomfortable but can be prevented with laxatives. Numbness in the hands can also occur with vincristine, as with many other drugs.

The time it takes to cure intermediate grade non–Hodgkin's lymphoma patients is usually several months. Additionally, a certain number of patients don't respond completely to the standard combination of the four chemotherapy agents, cyclophosphamide, vincristine, doxorubicin and prednisone, or the lymphoma returns at a later time. When Rituxan (rituximab) is routinely added to this combination, the chance of cure improves. Protocols using combinations of other second-line drugs are also available. These can be combined with stem cell bone marrow transplants to further improve chances of survival.

Mike: Continued Treatment Brought about a Positive Outcome

At the age of 39, Mike knew cancer all too well. Many in his family had suffered from the disease, including his mother, father, and brother. His brother developed a metastatic colon cancer at the age of 45. When Mike developed an intermediate grade lymphoma, he hoped that he would be one of the lucky ones cured by the standard combination chemotherapy. Although he was disappointed when his lymphoma returned, he continued to seek out other options. The disease returned shortly after he stopped the first set of six chemotherapy cycles. Undaunted, he agreed to treatment with second-line agents. The plan was to once again go through enough treatments so that he would achieve another remission. But instead of stopping as he had done the first time, he would go on for further therapy. The clinical trial that he was enrolled in not only involved a stem cell bone marrow transplant, but it also involved radiation therapy with a protracted period of therapy with an unapproved, experimental biological agent called IL-2.

Mike's lymphoma has been in remission for ten years now. We have continued to carefully follow him. After so such time, he is more likely to develop yet another type of cancer than to have his lymphoma return. Although he has developed numerous colon polyps, through close surveillance, he has not developed any new cancers.

MYELODYSPLASIA

Myelodysplasia is a blood disorder that is best thought of as a pre-leukemia condition. While it may occur at younger ages, it is generally thought of as a disease of elderly people. As we age, the chromosomes in our blood cells gradually become less and less stable, and our bodies become less competent in repairing accumulated DNA damage. This effect can occur in all of our body's cells. Over time, in some people, white blood cells morph into slowly growing preleukemic cells. This has the effect of reducing the normal blood counts and making a person anemic. It may also lower white blood cell and platelet count. As white blood count decreases, the immune system and the ability to resist infections begins to fail. When the platelet count decreases, you may see more bleeding in the urine, stool, or after surgery.

Myelodysplasia is often challenging to detect and to diagnose. The symptoms are vague and common. These include fatigue, anemia, weight loss, and frequent infections. The diagnosis is most easily made after an oncologist performs a procedure known as a bone marrow biopsy. This is where a small blood sample is removed from the pelvic bone of your hip. Most patients are able to tolerate the procedure well using various methods, such as good local anesthesia or sedatives. We find that patients are best able to tolerate the biopsy and recover quicker if they are simultaneously distracted, perhaps by music or a story. The bone marrow biopsy should be done by an experienced oncologist, so that it is performed quickly and with the least amount of pain. Your comfort should be paramount during a bone marrow biopsy. I have noticed that they're easier to tolerate when the physician is correctly trained and properly positioned. Many new molecular biological tests can be done on the bone marrow biopsy specimen. DNA studies are often needed to delineate among various blood diseases, such as the leukemias, lymphoma, myeloma, and myelodysplasia. Despite the newer DNA techniques, a diagnosis may not be clear cut. A series of bone marrow biopsies over time may be needed.

A person diagnosed with myelodysplasia has several treatment options. Younger patients may have the option of a bone marrow transplant. This means the bone marrow is donated by a stranger. Other options include supportive biologic drugs given by injection that try to increase the inadequate and low white blood and red blood cell count. These drugs don't treat the underlying condition, however. The low platelet count is more challenging to improve.

Various new chemotherapy drugs are available, including Dacogen (decitabine), Revlamid (lenalidomide), and Vidaza (azacytidine), some of which are given by vein and some of which are given by mouth. These drugs are able to increase the low blood counts by treating the underlying condition. They do this by actually acting on the malignant cells in the bone marrow. The specific clinical situation and the genetic makeup of the bone marrow biopsy results will help the oncologist determine which agents to consider. Because it is difficult to achieve a complete response, patients might be offered treatment with these drugs indefinitely. Treatments could stop when you either achieve a complete response or unfortunately progress to leukemia. It may be very hard to achieve a complete eradication of the abnormal cells in the bone marrow. It also may be difficult to know by the bone marrow and other tests if you are truly a complete responder.

MYELOMA

MULTIPLE MYELOMA

Multiple myeloma is a malignant growth of cells known as plasma cells. Normally found in the bone marrow, plasma cells usually produce the antibodies that help our immune system fight infections. When they become malignant, they can cause symptoms of bone pain, kidney failure, and infections. Myeloma can be very challenging to diagnose early. It takes a very astute primary care physician to be alert to the subtle laboratory test abnormalities in protein systems. More often patients arrive with a catastrophic problem, such as kidney failure, a bone fracture, or a life-threatening infection.

The myeloma cells grow in the bone marrow causing weakening of the bone. As they grow, they produce an excess of useless antibodies whose effect is to reduce the levels of normal helpful antibodies. Kidney failure occurs because these abnormal antibodies plug up the kidney system. Infections occur because the level of normal antibodies is too low. And bone fractures occur when the normal bone is weakened by too many myeloma cells. Neuropathy or nerve damage can also occur when these antibodies accumulate around and in the nerves. This neuropathy can cause numbness in the hands and feet. It may make it hard to detect subtle injuries to your feet and toes. (Patients with neuropathy should have their toenails trimmed by a podiatrist.)

The combination of these potentially catastrophic effects can be so extensive the patient may not be able to recover enough strength to receive the treatment. Usually myeloma is thought of as a systemic disease, which means that it is throughout the body. The diagnosis is made by a combination of blood tests on antibody types and levels and through a bone marrow biopsy. Various X-ray tests are also needed to examine for weakness or fractures in the bones. A fracture of many bones all at once occurs often. The infections may be very hard to treat without normal antibodies present.

The key to surviving myeloma is in getting diagnosed correctly and quickly. When this happens, it is necessary to rapidly make decisions about treatment. For many patients, complications from myeloma can best be avoided by starting chemotherapy quickly. At times, patients will come to the office in great need of pain relief. In an attempt to quickly relieve their suffering, some physicians will begin radiation to the most symptomatic areas. This may provide relief to them, but unfortunately it may also limit the amount and types of chemotherapy available to treat the remainder of the myeloma. Each time a different area of the body receives a series of radiation treatments, normal blood counts will lower. The treatments reduce the number of stem cells living in the bone marrow from which normal white blood cells grow.

Chelsea: Myeloma, but Still Playing Golf

Chelsea, age 70, prided herself on her golf game. She developed increasingly severe back pain, which became disabling, and she grew more and more fatigued over the months. Eventually, the pain grew to such an extent that she was bedridden. A low blood count led to worry about a possible blood disorder. The bone marrow sample was completely replaced with myeloma. An MRI of her spine was completed and explained the pain: Not only did she have myeloma affecting her entire spine, but she also had numerous fractures in it. Only when the spine breaks had been stabilized by a procedure known as a vertebroplasty did she feel relief. Vertebroplasty is a procedure in which bone cement is used to join together the broken pieces of the spine. This relieves the pain caused when the two pieces of bone rub up against each other; it also prevents further fractures.

Because she was older, she was a marginal candidate for a bone marrow transplant and was treated with standard chemotherapy mediation combinations by mouth and intravenously. After five years, Chelsea is comfortable and able to walk, shop, visit, and go about her usual activities. The only real problem is that because her myeloma in her spine had affected her height, her golf clubs are now too long. She is proud of her good, but short posture.

ADVANCED MYELOMA

If myeloma is extensive, the decision about whether to treat it is straightforward. But at times, with a much earlier form of the disease, observation is appropriate and can continue for many years. Monoclonal gammopathy of undetermined significance (MGUS) is a more limited form of a plasma cell disorder. Some, perhaps 25 percent of patients with this disease will eventually develop myeloma.

The chemotherapy regimens for myeloma involve oral medications as well as intravenous drugs. Several new advances have been made in the treatment of myeloma and have improved the chances of surviving. These include drugs such as Revlimid (lenalidomide) and Velcade (bortezomib) as well as Doxil (doxorubicin liposome injection),

Many, but not all, patients are able to achieve remission. In almost all cases, however, the myeloma eventually returns. Hopefully when it occurs, it is caught early before a catastrophic problem, such as fractures, kidney failure, or infections, happen. Some patients are offered consideration of bone marrow biopsies to improve their chances of continuing to be in remission.

Radiation therapy can be used to relieve the painful symptoms of myeloma affecting the bones. Its use should be limited and judicious as it will permanently affect the normal bone marrow reserve. The amount of radiation needed to treat myeloma is relatively modest.

CHRONIC LEUKEMIAS

Chronic Lymphocytic Leukemia (CLL)

Chronic lymphocytic leukemia is chronic leukemia of certain types of white blood cells known as lymphocytes. It may be found in the blood stream, bone marrow, lymph nodes, or all three. Many times, a routine blood test will find that the total white blood cell count is elevated. Of the several major types of white blood cells that make up our blood, the lymphocytes are the culprits that develop into these leukemic cells. While a patient may still have normal lymphocytes, if someone has CLL, he or she now has a population of malignant lymphocytes. Malignant CLL lymphocytes may also congregate in the lymph nodes. When this happens, the disease may be correctly called either CLL or a type of lymphoma known as small lymphocytic lymphoma. If CLL is associated with a swollen lymph gland that doesn't mean that the patient has a new type of cancer; it has just taken a new form.

Usually this leukemia is slow growing and may take months or years to develop before it requires treatment. Common symptoms for CLL are fatigue, weakness, swollen lymph nodes, and abnormal blood counts. The disease usually affects people in their sixties, seventies, and eighties. Many patients are found to have the disease during a hospital stay when being treated for an infection. Pneumonias and sinus infections are particularly common in CLL patients. While it is true that occasionally there is a need to wait until after pneumonia clears before treating CLL, it may be difficult to clear the pneumonia without special measures. These may include having pulmonary and infectious disease specialists help diagnose the particular type of pneumonia from which the patient is suffering. Those with CLL often come down with unusual types of infections. Other measures to help treat CLL may include infusions of antibodies known as gamma globulin. These can help recovery from an infection and prevent another one from developing. The level of antibodies in your system can be measured at regular intervals. Viral, fungal, or other unusual infections that are uncommon in normal people can cause quite a bit of illness if a patient has CLL. These include pneumonias from bugs such as pneumocystis carinii, cytomegalovirus (CMV), and staph.

Other problems also associated with CLL include a higher risk of developing blood clots, kidney complications, and the gradual onset of debilitating fatigue.

Because CLL is not a curable condition, treatment is sometimes delayed until after sufficient symptoms develop. These may include low blood counts, fatigue, and swollen lymph glands. Sometimes, the onset of these problems can be so gradual that it can be hard for you and your oncologist to decide when you need to be treated. The IV treatments available are usually quite effective and tolerable. These include both standard chemotherapy drugs, such as Fludara (fludarabine), Treanda (Bendamustine) or cyclophosphamide, as well as monoclonal antibodies directed against receptors on the leukemic cells. Campath (Alemtuzumab) and Rituxan (rituxumab) are examples of these antibodies.

Tolerating the short-term effects of the medications needed to treat CLL is often easier than dealing with the potential long-term complications from these same agents. That is, the patient may not notice immediate side effects, but the drugs may still be silently affecting his or her system. These include increasing the chance of developing other infections. Because the risk of infections affect all CLL patients, it is often a better strategy to treat the CLL and be monitored closely. Numerous ways to reduce the chance of infections exist. Some of them include taking prophylactic or preventative antibiotics and antiviral drugs, as well as vaccinations. The good news is that patients who are able to achieve a remission with these agents may sometimes be able to stay in remission for months or years.

A worrisome development is when the CLL is associated with numerous abnormalities in the DNA or chromosomes. Technology to discover DNA and bone marrow abnormalities in the lab is very highly sophisticated. If DNA contains these abnormalities, it generally means that patients will have a far more challenging time successfully treating CLL. It may require continuing on some form of effective treatment indefinitely if the CLL returns for this reason. Newer IV treatments may be able to partially overcome this DNA effect. Technology to discover DNA and bone marrow abnormalities in the lab is very highly sophisticated. At times the technology to diagnose the condition may be far more advanced than the treatment.

CHRONIC MYELOGENOUS LEUKEMIA (CML)

Chronic myelogenous leukemia is a cancer of white blood cells (known as myeloid or granulocytes.) These cells develop from normal white blood cells after a mutation occurs in two chromosomes. The biological abnormalities responsible for the development of this leukemia have been well known for years. This fact has helped the development of effective treatments. Unlike in the past, it is, therefore, rare to see a patient with advanced CML. While the term cure may still seem optimistic, newer agents are able to give most patients hope for long-term remissions.

Because these newer medications, including Gleevec (imatinib), are so remarkably useful, they have been able to reduce the number of CML patients who need to undergo risky allogenic bone marrow transplants. An allogenic transplant is one where the donor is someone other than you. While these transplants give the hope of cure, they also have substantial short-term risks, as well as long-term side effects that affect the patient's quality of life. Part of the effectiveness of the transplant comes from the substantial dose of chemotherapy that is administered immediately before the transplant. A second major part of the transplant, though, is from the new donor's white blood cells attacking leukemia cells.

When a patient undergoes a bone marrow transplant, the short-term risks of dying from either an infection or an acute reaction to the transplant are a major concern in the first several months. Patients may have had few, if any, symptoms from CML, but during the transplant they may become very ill. This happens despite newer methods to help reduce problems. These complications may depend on how close of a bone marrow match you have. The match process is a very detailed review of surface markers (called HLA or human leucocyte antigens) on the white blood cells. When a closely matched donor is selected, transplants are better tolerated. It has also been shown that transplant centers with more experience give patients the best chance of survival. Long-term survivors from allogenic bone marrow transplants also may have substantial side effects, including rejection, liver failure and infections.

The current treatments available for CML are likely to be effective for most patients for years. While resistance to these drugs does develop, second line agents such as Sprycel (dasatinib) and Tasigna (nilotinib) are also on the market. For most patients, starting treatment with oral agents and not a bone marrow transplant seems prudent. During the many years that they are responding to the currently available agents, other newer drugs may possibly be discovered. If choosing to undergo the transplant, any transplant-related problems, such as liver disease and rejection, could possibly be worse than the CML. Careful consideration and likely several consultations with the transplant physician and oncologist are needed before committing to an allogenic transplant. Depending on age, the quality of life might be better on Gleevec (imatinib) than it would be after a transplant.

ACUTE LEUKEMIA

Acute myeloid leukemia, a common type of acute leukemia, occurs in both the young and elderly. Initial symptoms include weakness due to anemia or infections such as pneumonias or sepsis. Some patients notice pain throughout the back or bone marrow in the spine and pelvis. The symptoms and problems develop very suddenly with acute leukemia, sometimes in just over a day or two.

Treatment for AML involves intensive chemotherapy usually administered as an inpatient. Complete eradication of the leukemia within the first several weeks is intended by using a combination of chemotherapy over a week's time. This intensive treatment results in very low blood counts for a week or two. During the time when counts are low, frequent transfusions and serious infections are a risk. Because of the very low blood counts, these infections can be life threatening. During the initial treatment, repeated bone marrow biopsies are done to check for remission or eradication of the leukemia.

AML can be a very difficult leukemia to treat, and it is not unusual for patients to need to be retreated after several weeks time. When this happens, patients may need to be hospitalized for a protracted period, often weeks. Lately, because of the worry that hospitalized patients will acquire resistant infections, some oncologists will treat some AML patients on an outpatient basis. This is safest to do when a motivated patient understands the warning signs of infection when the blood counts are low. Outpatient therapy also helps to avoid the depression that results from prolonged hospital stays.

Not all AML patients are alike. Some can have a more aggressive type of leukemia; it depends on the nature of the DNA changes. When these changes are associated with a poor prognosis, a bone marrow transplant may be considered. For some, the transplant could be recommended either immediately after a remission or eradication of the leukemia is seen. In others, this could be done when the leukemia returns.

AML occurs often in the elderly. In these circumstances, the treatment often needs to be individualized. Otherwise, healthy elderly patients may tolerate outpatient treatments better than expected. Also it may not be necessary to achieve complete remission; ongoing treatment that results in a stable condition might be acceptable.

Bill: Leukemia Masquerading as Trauma Pain

Bill was a 45–year-old white male who had been severely injured at work hurting his back and thigh one day. Continued pain led him to seek help from a variety of physicians. The history of the recent trauma diverted attention away from other potential causes of pain. Eventually, an MRI film detected an abnormal signal in the bones leading to the diagnosis of leukemia.

Other leukemia patients have been diagnosed as a result of symptoms as varied as abnormal bruises, bleeding gums, or meningitis

EMPOWER YOURSELF

These diseases—CLL, CML, myelodysplasia, and acute myeloid leukemia—all have long-term survivors and far more successful treatments than in the past. With the best available care, many patients survive with a good quality of life for years. But there are pitfalls, and better therapies are needed for those who don't respond.

WHAT'S NEXT

Although millions have received comfort and care in their last days through hospice, it has become a big business also. The next chapter will help you know whether it's right for you or someone you know.

Chapter 15

The Hospice Dilemma
Why It's Not Always the Answer

The care that hospices provide is universally and appropriately held in high esteem. By virtue of their impassioned service to the dying, their caregivers are held above reproach. But hospice is a business. Make that a very fast-growing, competitive, and profitable business. Discerning a patient's best interests, however, should be the priority. The person with cancer should be the center of the universe. Family members, friends, coworkers, bankers, and physicians are not.

In the past, patients died in the hospital, often after protracted stays. They frequently continued on treatments at the hospital and would die trying to survive. This happens less often now. Hospice has gained popularity as both a cost control means and as a way to prioritize comfort. Fewer patients currently die in hospitals, as there are many active hospice programs and Medicare and many insurers will pay for hospice. If you pursue treatment for cancer when it appears futile to your physicians, they may strongly encourage hospice.

A sign that an oncologist disagrees with a treatment decision can often be inferred from leading questions such as, *"You don't want to continue treatment, do you?"* *"Wouldn't you rather we focus on comforting measures?"* *"You don't want to give up do you?"*

Understand all that's involved when entering hospice. Many repercussions follow after the commitment is made. The decision needs to be made by the person with cancer. Don't let anyone force you to go to hospice. Similarly, don't let anyone prevent a patient from entering hospice if that is the choice. Also, the decision isn't irreversible. Some will change their minds. Patients *can* leave a hospice program after they've entered one.

Misunderstandings are common about hospice care. You may not know that if you are in hospice, you will probably not be allowed access to chemotherapy, radiation treatments, or hospitalization. It is also not home health care, which will be discussed below. That's a completely different service often given by the same agency.

WHAT IS HOSPICE?

To begin with, hospice is comforting care for a patient who is dying. Dying of anything. It doesn't matter if you are dying of cancer, AIDS, heart disease, or Alzheimer's disease. A few simple criteria need to be met, however. To qualify for the hospice Medicare benefit, physicians need to agree that the patient is likely to die in the next six months and that the condition is terminal. It is customary for aggressive medical treatments to be stopped and for only comforting measures to be continued. Morphine, oxygen, and suppositories for nausea are examples of comforting measures.

Contrary to what some believe, hospice is not teams of nurses and caregivers able to provide in-home care to anyone through their entire cancer treatment. It is not free care for the sick and elderly. It is terminal end-of-life care.

HOME HEALTH CARE

Home health care and hospice care are often distributed by the same agency. They are not, however, the same. Pay close attention to this detail. Home health care is temporary nursing care done in the home. It is often prescribed when healing from a medical condition, such as surgery, infection, or wound. It should not be confused with the terminal end-of-life care of hospice. At times, the home health staff may recommend hospice if they think a patient will be better served by that type of care.

HOSPICE CARE AT HOME OR AT A HOSPICE HOUSE

Hospice care can be given in the home, in a nursing home, or in a dedicated hospice center or house, but most hospice care is provided in the home. In this setting, the actual daily care is given mainly by the family and friends, not professionals. The hospice workers help to provide education, resources, and support. They will bring the suction machine, oxygen, hospital bed, and medications. They will then teach the support team how to use them. Generally, they don't do continuous care in the home.

In a dedicated hospice center or house, professional caregivers will attend to the patient if the family cannot. Different levels of care are available. If someone is actively dying, care and attention may be stepped up to ensure comfort. Various types of services are available for comfort. Relatively simple and inexpensive methods are employed first. The sick will be provided oxygen, bed rest, morphine, nausea medications, wound care, and the like. Comforting measures only.

WHAT TO ASK

Ask if the hospice has the needed supplies to care for the dying. If the dying is hospitalized and needs a high concentration of oxygen, make sure that the hospice is able to supply the same oxygen concentration. Let them know if you will be continuing to use medical devices, such as wound treatments or a specialty beds for bedsores.

If expensive medication to control symptoms is needed, make sure that they will provide them. For example, expensive injections are available to relieve the uncomfortable diarrhea due to slow growing bowel cancers known as carcinoid tumors. These injections often cost several thousand dollars each month. Will hospice provide them? Is the cancer patient allowed to have the epidural injections that have always helped the spine? (An epidural is when pain medication is injected nearby the spine to relieve discomfort.)

Will the person in hospice care be permitted to see other physicians? If you are admitted for lung cancer, can the patient continue to see an eye physician or lung doctor? Usually the hospice team of nurses, social workers, physician assistants, and physicians will decide how care will be administered. Ask if other doctors can be seen. At times this will be allowed as they are charged separately.

WHAT MAY NOT BE ALLOWED

Aggressive means of relieving suffering are generally not used in hospice settings. Even though radiation therapy and chemotherapy are intended to relieve pain, they are generally not allowed. Other more complex methods, such as epidural pain pumps and other pain injections, are also subject to the approval of the hospice agency. Usually cost is a prominent factor in the decision whether to pay for and administer such methods.

Common, inexpensive, uncomplicated, and comforting treatments that can be administered at the bedside by family members or nurses are the norm. Examples of these are pain relief medications and treatments such as morphine or anxiety medications to relieve the tension associated with terminal suffering. Experimental or costly treatments and clinic or hospital-based care are generally not done. Offering you hospitalization is also not expected. People shouldn't enroll in hospice if they expect to go to the hospital if their condition worsens. Occasionally, special circumstances, such as extensive wound care needs, require that patients receive their terminal care in the hospital. Another exception is when the patient's oxygen needs cannot be met or when it would be too uncomfortable for the patient to be moved into the hospice setting. You always have the option of changing your mind and leaving hospice. Usually, though, most patients can have their suffering relieved by an expert team in hospice.

WHEN SHOULD YOU CONSIDER HOSPICE?

Consider hospice care in several situations. If the cancer has stopped responding to doctors' prescriptions, has become resistant to all possible treatments, and the condition has weakened, hospice is a reasonable option. If the patient has a very resistant cancer that never responded to treatment, hospice might be an answer. In this phase of life, if the choice has been made not to not treat the cancer, hospice might be an answer.

If the patient is too weak and if he or she doesn't feel strong enough to go through treatment, consider this option. If the cumulative side effects of many treatments have weakened the patient, and he or she is unable to receive further mainstream care, then it is time to think about the hospice.

QUESTIONS A CANCER PATIENT SHOULD ASK
BEFORE ENTERING HOSPICE

Am I doing this for me or others?

Am I entering hospice because others don't want me to spend my nest egg on my health?

Am I doing this because I want to die comfortably and with dignity? Or has hospice been encouraged because my illness and death have become inconvenient and expensive for others?

Am I completely sure that my disease is untreatable? Do they have the correct diagnosis? Have I seen all the right specialists? Are there any appropriate off-label treatments that could be tried?

Am I giving up on the idea of treating my cancer because of depression? Is my cancer really untreatable or has my depression clouded my outlook? Have I sought treatment for my depression?

Am I entering hospice because an intimidating litany of drug side effects has terrified me and led me to not even try standard therapy?

Have I exhausted all opportunities to get financial help for treatments I assumed that I couldn't afford?

Am I considering hospice because I have no one to care for me? Even though a cancer might be responding to treatment, some consider hospice simply because they have no other options for placement.

WHAT IS NOT A GOOD REASON TO CONSIDER HOSPICE

If the patient is overwhelmed or if the family is overburdened by the care, possibilities to weigh before hospice include nursing home care, home health care, assisted living facilities, or VA medical centers. Caregiver fatigue syndrome hits everyone at some time. Those involved on a day-to-day basis with sitting with, driving, bathing, and putting out medicines, among other responsibilities, need a break. But that is not a good reason to enter hospice. Consider a respite program where for a brief time the cancer patient may be cared for in a facility while loved ones recharge batteries.

If there is trouble paying for care, possible solutions include applying for Medicaid, disability, or VA care. Look into the best options for using the remaining cash with a lawyer or social worker.

Being coerced by others to enroll in a hospice is not good. It needs to be a patient's idea.

Stopping effective treatment and considering hospice to save resources for survivors needs to be considered carefully. It is the patient's life and decision. Survivors always have the luxury of time to find ways to care for themselves and others. This is not always true for those with cancer. No one should enter hospice early to save survivors' money for a new consumer product. The hospice experience is better if patients go when they're ready.

Todd: Rescued from Hospice

Todd was a 71-year-old polio survivor who had been found to have a pancreatic mass. His family physician had hoped that a resection was possible and had sent him to the university hospital. At surgery, unfortunately, his pancreatic cancer could not be removed. Only a small sample for biopsy was taken. Todd's postoperative course was complicated by blood clots, pneumonia, and malnutrition. All of these had weakened him, and, at the university, it had been decided to enter him directly into the hospice program in his hometown. It was determined that his condition was too weak for chemotherapy or radiation treatments. He was sent to hospice untreated.

After he was in hospice for a week, he needed attention for an unrelated condition. I was called to evaluate him one Sunday on call. During our discussion about his injury, I learned about his pancreatic cancer story. I continued to visit him for several weeks. Over time, as he learned about the various options for treatment, his interest increased. With all of the complications surrounding his surgery, he had never seriously considered chemotherapy. He left the hospice center, received chemotherapy, regained his health, and was able to return to his community.

WHAT IS A GOOD HOSPICE EXPERIENCE?

Hospice services are provided by paid professionals, such as a physician medical director, nurses, and aides. Volunteers provide only nonskilled companion visits; families are provided education and materials that allow them to provide much of the care themselves. Those patients who have a favorable hospice experience share similar qualities, including:

- All those involved (family, friends, medical staff) universally accept that further therapy is unlikely to be helpful. There is no argument or discord about treatment choices.
- They accept the next phase of life. They embrace the hospice experience with as much energy as they would another project. You help those around you start the grief process. They engage in the hospice, grief, and loss process.
- Life work is full, if not done. Those with cancer have completed their life's work or at least given it a good start. She may be a 30-year-old mother, but she feels like she has started a family and passed on wisdom and part of her personality to a 5-year-old daughter.
- There is no depression. The cancer patients have a good attitude about hospice and are not dour. They dedicate themselves to a one day at a time attitude. They bring a smile and happiness to those around them, even in hospice. They are not bitter and depressed. They may even poke fun and joke about little things. People and family flock to see them.
- Patients are not forced by circumstances to be cared for somewhere they don't want to be. They have a plan, perhaps to donate property, land, or even their bodies when they pass. Occasionally, they will have arranged for themselves to be cared for in assisted living settings. One gentleman would bring a different memento into the office from home during each visit. Little by little, he was giving away pieces of art and memories that he had accumulated over the years. By the time he died, many members of the staff had cherished items with handwritten stories.
- They have accepted where they will be when they can't care for themselves. They turn little inconveniences into a positive. One patient had the offhand humor of deliberately releasing a little foul smelling gas

from his colostomy bag whenever a grumpy or less pleasant staff member was rude to him. One elderly man, bored by days in the hospital watching television, would laugh and deliberately switch the station to the breast examination channel showing a half naked woman whenever a staff member walked in the room.

This group has a legacy, a message, a style. A peace. People will remember their energy, embracing of life, and how they thought of others at this time.

Susan: A Celebration of Life

Susan was a 29-year-old single woman who, after an abnormal pap smear, had been diagnosed with cervical cancer three years earlier. While she was initially full of hope that her treatments would cure her, gradually her disease progressed. One day she found areas of cancer on her body that she knew were metastasis. Now she was sure she had a fatal disease, but she continued to go for her treatments, see her oncologist, and keep up her spirits. During this time, she met with old friends and family and kindly told them her story. With her strength and acceptance, she was able to tell others her sad news in a manner that put them at ease. If she was strong enough to accept her fate, others would be too. After several years though, it was time. She entered a hospice program and was cared for by her mother.

Susan prepared by encouraging her mother to see a psychologist to help her deal with the death of a daughter. She planned her own funeral, carefully orchestrating each part of the event, the burial plot placement, the music, the viewing, the drive to the cemetery. She even added sublime humor, choosing six old boyfriends (including yours truly) as pallbearers. She enjoyed several last trips to places that interested her. Her funeral was a celebration of her life and of life itself. She threw herself completely into the dying process, leaving those who knew her a great legacy.

POWER OF ATTORNEY, DNR, AND
OTHER IMPORTANT DOCUMENTS

There are several key documents that all cancer patients should have in place. The first is a living will, in which you can state preferences for certain medical procedures. A durable power of attorney for health care decisions, or a DPOA-HC, is also important. This document allows someone else to make health-care decisions for you when you're not able to. It is important that this person have a clear understanding of your wishes before assigning this responsibility, so discuss your views on end-of-life issues. This should be someone whose judgment you trust. You may not share the same outlook on life, but the person must understand and respect your views.

Both of these legal documents become effective only when you are incapacitated and no longer able to make decisions for yourself. You may rescind these documents at any time.

Another important form helps inform a medical team whether you wish to be resuscitated if the heart and lungs stop working. This form is known as a DNR form, which stands for Do Not Resuscitate. By signing this document, you are telling your physicians that when you start to pass away, you would rather die naturally than have aggressive measures taken. Without this document in place, the medical team will assume that you would like all possible measures taken. This may include intubation (where a tube is placed down the windpipe to help you breathe), ventilation (where a machine breathes for you), and cardioversion (where an electric shock is administered to help restore the normal heart rhythm.) Various intravenous medications are usually given as well. Some of these work to increase the blood pressure. For many patients with advanced cancer, it makes sense to sign a DNR form. If a condition has deteriorated to where you find yourself in a code blue procedure caused by cancer, it is rare that more can realistically be done. Commonly, patients find themselves in situations where all possible medical measures—everything short of a code blue and an aggressive ICU stay—makes the most sense.

MARKETING HOSPICE

In larger cities, many hospice agencies, both not-for-profit and for-profit, compete for the financially attractive business of services. Hospice services may be aggressively marketed and are usually paid for on a per diem basis by insurers and Medicare. Even though they have the best of intentions, this competition may result in unintended consequences.

When considering entrance to a hospice program, people need to do it on their own terms. They shouldn't grasp at last-minute options while their world is falling apart financially and physically. In the confusion of illness and with the rapid speed of events, people may be vulnerable. Before committing to a hospice, they should know exactly what services are going to be provided. They should be made aware ahead of time if any are to be limited.

Ellery: Too III for Hospice

Ellery was a 70-year-old woman who really had never engaged in modern medicine. She ignored the lump when her breast mass developed. Only after it rapidly enlarged and caused pain did she come in to be seen. Her breast cancer had spread to her lungs and liver. Unfortunately, her disease was responsive to treatment for only several months. Radiation therapy had been used to control the cancer on the chest wall. Late in her course she also developed a malodorous untreatable chest wall wound. To control it required complicated chronic wound care involving a wound vacuum and antibiotics. When she stopped active treatment, she considered hospice. Unfortunately, the local hospice would not pay for such complicated wound care. For that reason she decided to stay in the hospital until her death in order to remain comfortable around visitors.

The hospice team will assume that the diagnosis and medical care up to now have been correct and have followed the accepted standard of care. In other words, testing for treatable conditions is not the responsibility of the hospice. That job is up to you, your family physician, and your oncologist. The hospice's expertise is in offering comforting care, not oncology. Hospice is not going to double check whether or not your cancer should still be treated further or if you need a second or third opinion. Decisions such as these are very complicated for medical staff at times. For example, you may be suffering from a profoundly underactive thyroid and chronic leukemia. While the leukemia sounds ominous, the thyroid condition may be what is causing most of your problems and is very treatable.

YOUR DECISION OR SOMEONE ELSE'S?

For me, this is one of the most challenging sections of this book. As noted, don't let anyone be coerced into treatment decisions by friends, family members, or health care workers with an agenda different from yours. Even those very close to you could have a different agenda. For example, I have seen a wife, in futility, drag a weakened older husband out of bed, walk him around, and try to get him back to his truck-driving job. He clearly would have been better served by hospice.

I have also witnessed children refuse their parent's wishes to continue to receive treatment. I hope that their motivation was more charitable than the financial motives that appeared to be the case. At this time of crisis, when someone needs loved ones most, they disappoint and are less than charitable.

I don't pretend to know or understand all of the complex family dynamics at play during many family discussions. Time for cancer patients is both a burden and a luxury. Unlike those who may die suddenly, there is time to deliberate on life. They might take stock of life's accomplishments. The burden of time is when there have been wounds that haven't yet healed. Affairs, divorces, bad relationships, or words spoken in anger are revisited by loved ones. Children remember an alcoholic father. The time to make good on a long due promise to repair a relationship never comes.

An oncologist can tell something is wrong when discord, tension, and anger fill the air. At times I have been uncomfortable after hearing comments made by family members. In a rude, matter-of-fact manner, family members will ask questions that go beyond prognosis. *Is she really dying this time? How much time will it take? Can you tell me at the last minute, so I only need to make one trip? Can you not prolong things, since we're all here?* Clearly these questions reveal problems far beyond those on the surface.

Patients may also be the target of these up-front questions. *Have you made your funeral arrangements yet? We had plans for your money/land/ assets.*

In earlier chapters we discussed the importance of having a trusting relationship with a local oncologist. Talk it over with the oncologist or with the staff. The physician should be an independent guide to what is in the patient's best interest. If comfort measures are most important, do them. If the patient wants the option to continue treatment, it should be prioritized.

EMPOWER YOURSELF

Understand what hospice is and what it is not. Realize what care will be received in hospice, at home, or in the hospice house. Think about what makes a good hospice experience. And above all, understand that it is the cancer patient's decision and nobody else's.

WHAT'S NEXT

In the next chapter, we will look at the system in general and what can be done to make it work better. If we want, we can all help to make it better for each one of us.

Chapter 16

Hands-On Practical Help and Public Policy Advocacy
How You Can Make a Difference for Cancer Patients

The cancer system is like a hotel that is working just fine for the innkeeper but not the guests. Cancer patients should be the center of this universe—and they aren't. The major pharmaceutical companies, the local physician's offices, the neighborhood radiology center, the major not-for-profit cancer centers, the universities, the Medicare and Medicaid budgets, the insurance companies, and the for-profit home health and hospice agencies all have their own financial bottom lines to worry about. Their policies reflect this. Within the world of these organizations, their own financial health becomes priority one. In myriad subtle ways, the patient, is often shortchanged.

- Hospices won't accept someone as a patient if he or she is receiving chemotherapy designed to comfort and control symptoms. The high costs prevent these treatments from being a realistic option for improving comfort in most hospice situations.
- Corporate (or publicly owned) oncology offices promote physician use of those chemotherapy drug and supportive drugs that are the most profitable.

- Corporate oncology treatment paradigms favor less aggressive and thus less expensive adjuvant treatment options.
- Nursing homes select those patients who require the least amount of care, transportation, and staff time.
- Radiology services at various centers are compromised. These may include tests such as CAT scans, bone density checks, PET scans, or MRIs. In some radiology offices, the CAT scanner upgrade is delayed. It becomes more challenging to find radiologists who will generate reports useful in comparing old and new scans. Breast MRI tests may be available to some patients, based on the region and insurance, but not to others.
- Universities limit support of, and access to, clinical trials at their own centers which requires patients to drive a longer distance for research care.
- Hospitals develop programs that aggressively advocate for the right to hospice and comfort care instead of aggressively advocating for treatment.

PHARMACEUTICAL COMPANIES

The actions that pharmaceutical companies take also contributes to the patient being shortchanged.

- Drug companies stop supporting clinical trials that expand the uses of their drugs to less common cancers.
- Drug companies stop providing the support, information, and financial guarantees that allow patients the off-label use of their pharmaceutical agents. Some, but not all, drug companies will replace the drug in the physician's inventory if insurers don't eventually pay for a treatment. (Off-label treatment is when a chemotherapy drug, approved for one cancer, say colon cancer, is used to treat a second cancer, say lung cancer.)

INSURANCE COMPANIES

Insurers are a common stumbling block for patients to receive the care they need. It helps to have an advocate, preferably an oncologist who can argue knowledgably on a patient's behalf.

- Insurers start to limit payment for drugs unless the clinician strictly adheres to a study which led to FDA approval.
- Insurers assign meddlesome case managers to limit care for their benefit, not those of the patient.

FEDERAL PROGRAMS

Federal programs have so many intricacies and rules that the patient often gets overlooked. Elected officials should be one resource that can sometimes help you cut through the bureaucracy to quickly get the care the patient deserves.

- Federal programs, such as Medicaid and Medicare, delay updating and increasing payment for disability and for physician payments. As a result, patients become unable to afford to pay high spend-downs.
- Medicare pays for off-label treatments in some regions but not others.

CANCER CENTERS

Look carefully at the care you are receiving at the cancer centers. Your hometown oncologist should be available to advocate for you.

- Major cancer centers limit care to only on-site treatment resulting in higher travel costs to the patient.
- Major cancer centers limit care if the patient is from out of the area.

Christopher: Not a Hospice Priority

Christopher lived nearby about an hour's drive away and was ready to consider hospice in his hometown. He had battled his throat cancer for years, only to be left with terrible pain that persisted despite endless numbers of morphine pumps and other devices. He had waffled back and forth about his decision to stop his chemotherapy. He was only receiving marginal benefit from it. For a week or two after he received it, the mass would shrink slightly and be less painful. But his weight had slipped, and Christopher was often bedridden. Between the growing tumor and the effects of previous surgeries and radiation, his appearance was sorrowful. We all knew that he would not be allowed to continue his chemotherapy treatments when he was in a hospice program. Our social worker had taken the time over several months to develop a relationship with him. She had been concerned that the nursing home he had found himself in was poorly able to meet his end-of-life needs. Eventually a compromise plan was worked out where he would get his chemotherapy treatment, then later that same day travel to the hospice to look over the facilities. If he liked the place and people, he would stay for a two-week trial period. He agreed. Early in the day, the hospice facility had agreed to set up the tour and meeting, but when the time came to see the facility, the social worker was told not to bring him because, "We're having a really big holiday staff party." Christopher was sent back to the nursing home. I'm sure that the staff members being recognized at the party had years of devoted service to patients in hospice. But, the patient needs to be the focus, not anyone or anything else. At this time of life when there is suffering, it's time to be the center of the universe.

AGGRESSIVE OR ALTERNATIVE TREATMENT OPTIONS

Unless all of these above organizations—hospice, public corporations, physicians offices, hospitals—are financially sound, they can't stay in business. Providing and advocating for cancer treatment is how they make money. In the above examples, and in hundreds of similar ways, financial incentives such as these limit the chances of having cancer treated and cured. Far more incentives in the system exist to limit and stop care than to promote and extend it. The current system almost requires the patient to develop a relationship with a benevolent oncologist and group willing to advocate on his or her behalf if aggressive treatment is to be pursued.

Many more patients exist who want to have this option than there are oncologists who are willing to provide such choices. At some point, many will hear the unfortunate news that there is nothing else that can be done.

This is very hard to accept. Even very ill patients will seek out other treatment possibilities. This is their right. Often it is psychologically easier to keep trying. There is a great need in the cancer treatment arena for people who don't want to accept or who can't accept their fate. These patients resist stopping treatment. Part of the pressure to continue therapy is based on misunderstanding and a lack of faith in conventional therapy. Because there are so many myths and so much misinformation about cancer, a revamped education program would be useful to help educate the public about conventional appropriate treatment.

Ideally this need would best be filled by enrolling in appropriate research trials that run a small but real chance of helping patients and a greater chance of aiding others by improving understanding. In this way, they'll continue to be offered a chance of improvement within the safety of a monitored study. But the clinical trial world is rigid; it lacks compassion and understanding. There are rules and timetables and deadlines. No, you can't delay treatment for your grandson's wedding. No, we can't allow that particular nausea medication to be given.

Many resist this regimented end-of-life plan and instead run to the pleasant neighborhood alternative or natural medicine shop. These other, less conventional organizations, step in and fill this extremely profitable niche. Well-intentioned people work and serve in this alternative marketplace with little knowledge of whether any real help is being sold. When you move outside the world of conventional medicine, you lose all of the protections you expect from FDA-approved drugs. For all of its tardiness and limitations, the painfully slow drug development process does prioritize safety.

In addition to the large alternative herbal therapy market, other organizations offer to serve when someone doesn't wish to stop treatment. These include the elaborate boutique specialists' offices, as well as hybrid offices and hospitals that combine both alternative and standard treatment facilities. Often little is gained at these facilities other than style points and filling the hope void left when other physicians give an overly blunt, pessimistic, formal clinical oncology assessment. Free massages, ornate offices, airport valets, and gourmet food are all blatant attempts at marketing. They help to soften the message and relive the guilt of survivors, but in the end do little to help.

The alternative drug market has been permitted to exist with limited oversight for so long that it has taken on a life of its own. Despite the lack of substantive data to justify its use, and with a bewildering array of different products to select from, the alternative therapy market has continued to grow. It is easy for herbal therapies to appear useful when diseases that are slow to change and often require no therapy at all are being treated. Its magnitude reflects the failure of conventional medicine to provide an answer when someone chooses to refuse to give up and desires to keep trying something.

Just as it is imperative that the right to stop therapy be respected, it is important to respect the right to continue to seek appropriate treatment. Wherever you live, whatever the insurance. These options must be permitted to expand the universe of acceptable therapies. If vast numbers of patients are willing to submit to treatment with fish cartilage or special teas, certainly the numbers exist to enroll in more helpful but better administered, less costly, and more convenient clinical trials.

Delilah: Turned Away at the Alternative Shop

Delilah, age 55, hadn't needed to see a physician since the birth of her now 35-year-old son. She prided herself on her good health and, despite a lack of regular exercise, was usually strong and worked on her husband's farm with him from sunup to well after dark. For several months she had been having increasing fatigue and occasional back pain. It worsened despite trying many over-the-counter potions, creams, and gels. She became increasingly desperate and turned for advice to an alternative therapy center. She was not at all inclined to seek the advice of a physician. By the time she reached the center, she was essentially bedridden and needed a wheelchair. While she could answer many questions, she tired easily. The staff at the center appreciated how ill she actually was and that she was unlikely at this late stage to benefit from therapy. They prudently ran a few routine lab tests and referred her to an appropriate physician.

Delilah had a critically high calcium level brought on by an advanced case of multiple myeloma, a blood cancer. She was near comatose. By delaying a medical evaluation, she risked kidney failure, fractured bones in her spine, paralysis, and infections. While her conventional chemotherapy treatments were not guaranteed to succeed, there was essentially zero chance for the alternative therapies to treat her condition at this late stage. The good health she had enjoyed for so many years was fortuitous, but was probably unrelated to any potions or concoctions in which she invested. Her tardiness in seeking attention by the physicians who could help her almost led her to snatch defeat from the jaws of victory.

After a several week stay in the intensive care unit, she was able to return home to the family farm. She continues on treatment regularly and is continuing to respond.

FEDERAL POLICY PROBLEMS

Endless current federal policies have had dramatic, far-reaching, unpleasant, and unfortunate effects on the cancer system. As you may suspect, these effects are not always fair. Some of the problems are listed below.

- Why are the Federal dollars used to develop new treatments focused on mostly common cancers, many of which already have new treatments available?
- Why are screening and prevention studies very limited, not universally available, and underfunded?
- Why are research studies run in a way that effectively limits the enrollment of certain groups, especially people from rural areas, the poor, and minority populations?
- In the case of rare cancers, why does Medicare restrict oncologists to using only those chemotherapy drugs proven useful in clinical trials when no such studies will ever exist within the current system for such rare diseases?
- Why is Medicare reimbursement for drug expenses effectively better for larger clinics than it is for smaller oncology offices?
- Why are Medicare patients required to come into the office for daily blood product support medications rather than more conveniently self-injecting themselves at home?
- Why isn't an oncologist's judgment considered when a patient needs therapy for situations that couldn't possibly have been previously re-

searched, and therefore, don't have appropriate treatment guidelines? These situations occur hundreds of times a day, such as when you need chemotherapy for two advanced malignancies simultaneously. Other similar situations are when a person is diagnosed with a treatable cancer, such as a small cell lung cancer or a lymphoma that has caused just enough liver or kidney failure to prevent someone from being eligible for most research studies. Not all problems can be researched; your oncologist's advice is essential.

- If you have a very rare type of cancer, such as a malignant hemeangioendothelioma, adrenal cortical cancer, or castlemen's disease, why aren't easily administered clinical trials close to home available anywhere in America? Without such studies, only painfully slow progress will ever be made in the treatment of these rare tumors. Realistically, only a small percentage of patients with these cancers will be able to travel to large centers for the available research studies.

- Why is it effectively prohibited for community physicians to use the tremendous assets of the pharmaceutical companies to facilitate publishing reports when such rare tumors are successfully treated off label? Without such access to this information, valuable information will never be accessible to the public.

- Why aren't pharmaceutical companies protected from the fear of liability when researching treatment options for uniformly fatal cancers that tragically take the lives of young people? The research into the usefulness of new biological drugs for the treatment of brain tumors is such an example. Without such protection, "the system" is far more comfortable with patient's dying of brain cancer than with being treated, with a much smaller risk of dying, from a new treatment. It is understood that drug companies will naturally fear the small but present risk of severe side effects that can turn a tragic cancer death into a financial judgment against the company. For this reason, the drug development and approval process slows to a glacial speed, requiring endless numbers of studies documenting ever more minute details before these drugs are released to help those who are dying from lack of access.

Other problems unnecessarily generated by the federal bureaucratic oversight include:

- When every clinical medical lab is already certified by Medicare, why is extra expense being spent duplicating this work by certifying each lab for each research study?
- Why are the calculations for estimating the living expenses for cancer patients on Medicaid so onerous? Who is supposed to advocate for the poor by updating the monthly living expense calculations known as the spend-down rate for Medicaid patients?
- Why does Medicare have a regional system to approve treatments rather than a national one? Are the cancers in patients in one state different from those in another state?
- Why are there a handful of research hospitals across the country exempt from the standard Medicare DRG system that sets payments for inpatient care expenses?
- Why does Medicare make dramatic changes in reimbursement for oncology services rapidly and without an opportunity for the physicians and the market to adapt and make appropriate changes?

Mike: A Victim of Bureaucratic Inertia

Theresa and Mike have been visiting our clinic for months. She had been devoted to him for the 50-odd years of their marriage and was committed to helping him in his effort to survive cancer. They accepted with ease the requirement that, when needed, she would drive him to the office for his shots. (We didn't tell them that the younger patients with third party payers could self-inject at home.) She had grown tired one day and hit an ambulance when driving him to the clinic. Although they both survived the accident, he was hospitalized and required substantial medical attention.

There is absolutely no reason other than bureaucratic inertia for Medicare's requirement that for certain drugs are only reimbursed if given in the office.

These and many similar problems plague cancer patients. It is understood that nothing was ever invented and perfected on the same day. Every cancer patient, friend, or family member has a stake in this complex system. In its goals to treat patients, it is a flawed system, and its flaws have caused the needless loss of lives.

WHOM TO CALL TO HELP CHANGE THE SYSTEM?

Advocacy groups ? Your congressperson? Your local Medicare representative? Your local Medicare office? Amgen? Your hospital? No, I don't know either. Nobody knows. The system is a many-headed hydra that is beyond anyone's control. Large amount of Federal and state funds as well as large amount of money from insurers and individuals are involved.

Try to call your congressperson, and you eventually get a bureaucratic response long after it might have been helpful in the clinic. Their broad strokes that affect big policy decisions are of little help day to day. Yet an enormous amount of money flows through congress. Research dollars, Medicare, and disability funds all start here. Other revenues are paid with state funds but are mandated at the federal level. With good intentions, lawmakers have tried their best to both protect the interests of the taxpaying public and serve those suffering from cancer. They have sought the advice of experts at various universities and think tanks. Few times if ever, however, is advice sought from physicians who have the most firsthand experience dealing with real-life problems. The difficulty starts when the laws are turned into regulations that federal and other offices administer. You can be flexible, bureaucracies can't. The people who work in these offices have a tremendous interest in carefully adhering to the letter of the law. How would it benefit them if they try to be flexible and understand a personal situation? Don't expect it.

Advocacy groups often fruitlessly compete with each other in efforts to obtain revenue for their individual programs and constituents. Changes are based on advice from similar professional experts. As they become further and further removed from the patients for whom they are advocating, the message becomes less relevant. The cancer advocacy movement has long been professional and polite. It is also, as you can see, less than perfect in helping to effect change that helps you, the patient, day to day. Fundraising efforts of local and national chapters of these groups need to earmark a certain amount of money for projects that recognize the donors but do little to actually help the cancer patient. Elaborate centers built with such funds may help only to receive this recognition, while actual hands-on help, such as in-home care or help with finding funds for medical expenses, is difficult to find.

Drug companies lack a cohesive industry group with which to organize and spread their message. Many similar industries have developed organizations found to be useful to members. The oncology pharmaceutical companies, however, have hurt themselves by not having such an organization and spokesperson. By dealing with the Federal institutions separately, they compromise their chances to effect change. By having such an organization made up of companies that produce and market chemotherapy pharmaceuticals, they would start to get things done. Such change might even be able to work toward advocating better access to all patients at all steps in the drug development process. Another change that such an organization might strive for is to help the general public understand the cancer treatment process as a whole and the great advances that have been made in the last 25 years. As it is now, the piecemeal marketing gives all of us a very disjointed view of cancer treatment. The drug companies are the only ones that have the budget to produce such a campaign.

Professional oncology organizations have had limited roles in effecting real change in the day-to-day problems of the oncologist's practice. The status quo is largely maintained, leading to continued inconveniences for many patients and caregivers.

Clinical trials need to be organized to prioritize the utmost convenience of the patients. At times, some of these studies appear to reinforce the marketing of what are protected franchises. When a patient asks me, "Why can't I receive this treatment closer to home?," I have no answer. When persistent inquiries are made, the drug company sponsor says it is the rule of the cooperative group, which blames the large cancer center organization regulations, which notes the requirements of the FDA, which notes institutional review board (or IRB) patient safety concerns. . . . In fact, other than simply protecting bureaucratic fiefdoms and assigning liability concerns, there is no real reason why most patients can't be treated on most clinical trials most of the time at the closest oncology office. Of course, for many reasons, including limiting travel costs, limiting travel safety concerns, and improving quality of life, by being at home, patients may find the option of nearby treatment desirable. After the first several treatments at the primary research institution, follow-up therapy could be done at the office as close to home as possible. Data and information could be obtained from the office, and appropriate payment made to the primary oncologist office for its services.

If a comprehensive organization that included drug companies, advocacy groups, and oncologist were to exist, real change might occur. The attitude would need to be a proactive, assertive one that is emboldened in its efforts to advocate for better lives for cancer patients. In an effort to ensure a proactive patient-centered approach, the board of such an organization should include patients, caregivers, and practicing oncologists. Such a group could announce and market to the general public the effectiveness of conventional treatments, as well as describe the usefulness of clinical studies. Hopefully this could limit the vast numbers of patients who decline effective treatments with known side effect profiles for unstudied and impure alternatives.

Bake sales of doughnuts decorated with multicolor bows or fun run exercises are not to be mistaken for activities that are directly helping cancer patients. Instead, they help the participants far more than they do the cancer patient. Rarely will our frivolous cancer fundraising—where marketing efforts are aimed at selling daffodils, t-shirts, or ball caps—affect which drugs are directly available to cancer patients. These efforts are not page one, they are extras, or fluff.

Sufficient bureaucracy exists to defend the entrenched fiefdoms in the current system to render such timid efforts impotent at providing effective advocacy help. The early years of the HIV movement taught us that real change, which aggressively advocates for the patient, doesn't occur without media involvement and risk. By challenging those who are willing to erect roadblocks in the path of ill cancer patients, we will make a difference. A bit of our time may be involved. This type of advocacy is not comfortable; it isn't there for us but for the patient. It involves a little ingenuity. It is spontaneous. There is a risk of exposure, and maybe even of bail. But it is far more effective at producing real change, and cancer patients deserve it.

Leo: Promises Not Kept

Leo, a 77-year-old veteran (and a smoker), had served his country in the armed services. His multiple myeloma treatment was complicated by his smoking, his lack of family support, his multiple other medical problems, and his modest means. Most drugs were too costly for him; he relied solely on the government hospital for prescriptions. While he was eligible for care provided by the government, it wasn't made very user friendly. He would need to make several long, tiring, and expensive (for him) trips to the government facility before the system would possibly approve the latest oral drugs. The prescription and recommendation by his community oncologist wasn't sufficient. The drug was repeatedly denied even though he jumped through hoops, because the determination as to whether an agent is paid for by the government system is regional.

Leo had several strikes against him, including some, like smoking, that he did to himself. But the ones added by a government bureaucracy seemed the cruelest. He had risked his life serving his country. Late in the course of his illness, a foundation graciously agreed to fund the drug. The government hospital never did. By delaying his access to the latest approved therapy, the government had kept Leo from benefiting from years of research and drug development. Why do the research if access will be denied?

By relying solely on the government hospital for prescriptions and by smoking, Leo needlessly put himself in a risky situation. Eventually, after his death, an ad-hoc group of his physicians, foundation advocates, and pharmaceutical company personnel have begun to call those responsible to the carpet by pointing out to the appropriate authorities how unfairly Leo was treated.

WHAT CAN YOU DO: PRACTICAL STEPS

While all of the others are deliberating about policy and system-wide problems, you can make a big difference right now.

- Whether you are a cancer survivor, patient, or family member, practical hands-on help is always needed. Focus on activities that directly help individuals suffering with cancer. These situations may initially be more uncomfortable as they involve getting to know another person in a human way. Many of us worry about feeling an emotional loss when the one that we are helping has a chance of dying. But many times by remembering the times that we have had with them, our own lives become more fulfilled. We see the world in a different way. Here are a few suggestions that describe the real help that many need today. Don't be scared. Just do it.

Be supportive. Don't be negative. Even when the situation looks grim, and death may be imminent, there is always something positive to say, "They are doing a good job of controlling your pain, Joe, aren't they?" or "You have been an inspiration to others with how you have put up with this disease."

- Negative statements don't help. Insistently asking the patient again and again, "Do you understand that you are going to die?" for a tenth time is negative, but people do it all of the time. So is, "Are you ready to die?" Wait for them to open up and ask about these things first. Everyone faces their own mortality in different ways. Theirs may be worlds different than the way in which you would handle your situation. That's okay. Accept the difference. It's their time, not yours.

- It helps to keep the best attitude that you can. One patient Joey had an advanced kidney cancer that spread to his lungs, liver, lymph nodes, and spine. His attitude was always great. He would arrive with a mood and outlook better than ours. Only he's the one who had the metastatic cancer. "I'm going to wear this uncomfortable spine brace all day and night," he said about a very unwieldy spine brace. "That way if I slip and fall and go paralyzed, at least I can say that I tried my best."

His attitude toward asking about his prognosis and about how long he had to live was, "No time lines. That's giving up. I want to take each day as it comes."

- Transportation is one of the biggest day-to-day needs that patients have. To get someone to an oncologist almost always requires another in the family to take at least a half-day off from work. While this may seem imperative at the time of diagnosis, when there is a great deal of unknown and panic, gradually this changes. Work and other responsibilities become more important. Liability concerns limit the number of institutions that are willing to take on this responsibility. Patients may not be able to safely drive themselves because of the cancer or treatment-related fatigue. Those who are able to help drive others to and from their treatments and appointments are greatly appreciated. They often note how rewarding it is for them. Also, if you allow someone else to drive you to the oncologist, patients feel less like they are burdening their families. This kind of help also allows safe transport with dignity (without having to go through the painful process of taking away someone's driving license when they become too weak to drive.)

• Medical bills and other financial concerns are challenging to deal with when you feel well. When you are sick, they can be a nightmare. Having limited resources can make matters even worse. On top of all this, cancer is very democratic and affects people from all walks of life. This includes the well educated and sophisticated, as well as those with more limited educations and abilities. It is the latter groups that often find themselves needlessly sent into the collections line. Helping to explain programs, bills, and policies can be very useful. Even just filling out forms requesting help can be daunting for many. The single or depressed person is particularly at risk to run into financial trouble that can affect treatment. Going to the business office, explaining forms, organizing forms, and making phone calls all helps. You can do this while you wait if you are driving her to the appointment. If you live a distance away, you can also help by trying to help find resources that the patient needs. This may include safer or more affordable housing or finding organizations that help with travel expenses, medical expenses, or lodging. From a distance, you may also be able to advocate for the patient to get help with expenses associated with medications and expensive drugs. Each individual drug that the patient needs help with requires its own series of forms to be completed. Finding, compiling, arranging, and completing these forms all takes time and requires help.

• Sitting with cancer patients at home, at hospice, or during their treatments makes a huge difference. For a while it removes them from the current situation. They become engrossed in hearing about your trip to Rome or new grandbaby. Stories that they tell you about their life, their marriage, their war experiences, and family all serve to help to wrap up their lives. Discussing the ordinary routine of life, such as the weather and the news, also relieves the suffering and passes the time more pleasantly. By merely being with someone in his home, you can motivate him to help himself by assisting him with walking or exercise. You also might notice little items around the home that may be unsafe. These could include extension cords or throw rugs. Bundles of stuff left on stairs that a patient might trip on also need to be removed. Many elderly people use a type of walking in their home known informally as "furniture walking," where they hang on to one piece of furniture after another as they move about the home. Watch them and try to make the environment safer.

• Getting essentials and running errands helps also. Having cancer or taking treatments is almost a full-time job. When you feel sick is not exactly the time when you want or are able to start running around town on errands. These include going to the pharmacy on numerous trips and bringing records to the physician's office, the hospital, the social security disability office, the social worker, and others. Getting the financial help that the cancer patient needs requires a great deal of paperwork. I have problems organizing this paperwork on a good day. You also might help by getting medical supplies and adaptive equipment. A ramp so that a wheelchair can be brought into the home is a common need. Getting wheelchairs and devices so that the patient can bathe safely is also important. So are grab bars for the bath and hand wands for the showerhead. Sometimes a home will have to be reorganized for a walker or wheelchair The ill cancer patient may need groceries from a variety of places to fill a need for food that tastes different. Although the usual favorites may no longer appeal to the patient, perhaps the Tandori chicken from that Indian restaurant across town tastes great. Go get him some.

• You may also offer to help or find help with the responsibilities that the patient has committed to. Otherwise, she might stop treatment to fill the commitments previously agreed to.

"I can't take chemotherapy or radiation treatment now because I need to help care for my parents."

• Helping others to find useful available clinical trials, physicians, and other information may also be a hands-on type of service that you can do. Often Web-based resources, as well as the resources from your primary oncologist, can help. At times, patients need help making phone calls as well as organizing, sending, and copying medical files and other information.

All of the above and more are the many ways you can directly or indirectly assist cancer patients. Don't be wary or intimidated. Don't be scared off by fears of emotional loss or potential liability. Help!

Paula and Lori: Who Was Involved?

Paula, a 45-year-old old attorney, well known in social circles, had been very successful in her law practice. She enjoyed dressing up and attending benefit auctions while visiting with friends. At tax time, she remembered the several thousand dollars a year she would donate to cancer and other charities. But her involvement was limited. She was only an attendee. She thought that by donating an evening of her time and some money, she was helping cancer patients.

Lori was also another successful attorney. She attended social functions because she had to, not because she wanted to. She would rather work or meet with people one on one. She networked, volunteered herself for committees, and got involved. When a physician's office called about a patient who needed help writing a letter to an insurer or employer, she would volunteer to help. She even took time to go on the barnstorming tour to Washington, DC, one year. She was hands on.

Having elderly parents to care for doesn't change the fact that your own cancer is at risk to recur and that you need to go through your own treatment. Patients will look for almost any reason to not receive recommended treatments. If you can help, find others to take over these responsibilities so that the patient gets his or her own needed treatments.

Bill: Proactive Friends

Bill, a 47-year-old farmer, was diagnosed with breast cancer. He had always been athletic and had many friends. His wife worked for the Federal government and provided the family with excellent insurance. Even though he had always wanted to be aggressive with his cancer treatment, about five years after his diagnosis, his doctors discovered spread of his cancer to a single site in the liver. They hoped that by surgically removing the liver metastasis and then by treating him with chemotherapy, a long-term remission might still be possible. Bill tolerated his treatments well and had an infectious and aggressive spirit. After his treatments stopped, he had regular follow-ups with CAT scans and lab tests. The insurance company, however, balked at paying for the more sensitive (and expensive) PET scans. Once again several years later, his cancer showed up on a lab test and CAT scan of his liver. His doctors again hoped that this was an isolated area of spread. If it was, perhaps another attempt at removing it by surgery or some newer local treatment could be considered. His previous liver operations had made his CAT scans hard to interpret. Unfortunately, his insurance would not cover the important PET scan.

After Bill lamented his woes to his compadres over some brewskies one evening, they offered to help. One of his friends knew a relative of the anchorman at a local TV station. Several phone calls later, and a human interest story was in the works. Another friend offered to intervene by calling the insurance commissioner. Ultimately, Bill's friends were able to get the PET scan paid for by his insurance where the doctors and others had failed for years.

Bill enjoyed real help in a hands-on manner by friends who weren't afraid to intervene. Proactive help that makes a difference in someone's care sends a message of love that fun runs don't.

A POSITIVE OUTLOOK

With an understanding of how to navigate the cancer system, cancer patients and their loved ones can make better use of all available resources . Although visits to out-of-town experts may be necessary, working and bonding with the oncology team close to home will greatly improve chances of survival.

In addition, families and supporter groups are better able to help to provice real down-to-earth help. Federal programs, state insurance programs, and helpful foundations are also available. Remember that many great oncology professionals are willing to help. These men and women devote their lives and energy to cancer patient care. New drugs, new surgical and radiation techniques, new support, and advocacy programs are always being developed..

The many small successes that have happened in cancer research over the last thirty years are now coming together. The treatment of cancer is far more successful than most people believe. See your oncologist. Listen, talk, and develop a bond.

Appendix

50 Questions and Answers
What My Patients Ask

1. Will I get sick and vomit?

    Probably not if you pay attention to your oncologist's instructions. The newer antinausea medications may be costly, but they do work well. Pay attention to treating anxiety, constipation, and reflux.

2. Should I take this herbal supplement that my cousin is selling?

    No. Not unless your oncologist approves. It is doubtful that there will be good clinical trials demonstrating that it is useful, and it could be harmful.

3. What is my prognosis?

    Good question. You need to ask your oncologist. It may take him some time to sort out your stage and the nature of your cancer. Likely it is better than you think.

4. Can I work?

    Ask your surgeon or oncologist. For the first several weeks after surgery, you may need to limit lifting, and this could affect your work. If you work as a psychologist, you can probably return to work sooner than if you are a heavy equipment operator.

5. How much will these treatments cost?

    Likely more than you think. Make a budget and plan on meeting your deductible each year. Your worry should only be about getting treatment for your cancer. Let others worry about the big picture of controlling health care costs.

6. Should I go to the big cancer center 10 hours away?

    It depends on the nature of your cancer, your health and ability to travel, and your ability to pay the travel and other expenses. For most cancers, you should be able to receive your care at home. If you need reassurance or if you have an unusual situation or cancer, you might ask your oncologist to help you find a physician at the big center. But don't travel 12 hours just to see an expert's physician assistant.

7. Will I lose my hair?

    Probably not, but with certain drugs, it is expected. But it is not a good idea to let fear of hair loss drive your treatment decisions.

8. Should I have radiation therapy or chemotherapy?

    It depends on the type of cancer you have and on a number of other factors. This is a good question to ask your oncologist. If he or she gives you a choice between the two, pick the one with the fewest long-term side effects. Chemotherapy usually has different and often fewer long-term side effects.

9. Do I have to keep taking this drug?

    Unless your oncologist asks you to stop, many cancer drugs, such as hormone drugs for breast and prostate cancer, are taken indefinitely. Other oral chemotherapy drugs are taken on a specific schedule. Make sure you have a good understanding of the schedule.

10. Does my mom or dad really understand the prognosis?

    They probably have been told repeatedly but haven't internalized the information. It may need to be told to them in a different manner so that they can understand. Alternatively they may simply be in denial and may not be ready to hear bad news.

11. Why should I take chemotherapy when everyone knows that it has side effects? The herbals treat cancer naturally and have no side effects.

All effective cancer treatments will have side effects. "Natural" treatments are permitted to make any claims, some outlandish. Approved treatments given by your oncologist have well-known side effects and well-known benefits. The side effects of chemotherapy may be limited by good patient education. Weekly chemotherapy treatments are also an option that limit side effects.

12. Is it true that a surgeon cutting into a cancer makes it spread?

No. Cancers spread all on their own, and this is unaffected by surgery. Frequently though, the preoperative CAT scans and other tests can tremendously underestimate the amount of cancer.

13. How did I get this cancer?

Statistically the most likely reasons are smoking, a strong family tendency to get cancer, and significant exposure to environmental agents such as asbestos, radiation, or herbicides. For most cancers, no reason is found.

14. I only smoke five or ten cigarettes a day. Is that bad?

Yes. Any cigarette smoking will affect your cancer treatment. It not only will reduce your chance of responding to your treatment, but it will also increase your chance of developing a second cancer.

15. Do CAT scans cause cancer?

For most cancer patients, CAT scans are a very useful test and are crucial to your oncologist's treatment decisions. The amount of radiation that you might be exposed to with each CAT scan is very small. But to be safe, for younger patients, it may be wise to use only the minimum number of CAT scans necessary.

16. Do I need to change my diet?

Usually not, unless your oncologist recommends that you change. Limiting salt intake is common. Most people who ask this question want to know if a different diet will help limit the growth of their cancer. Unfortunately, it won't.

17. I've been trying to lose weight. Is that good?

NO. Weight loss is a very, very bad sign. Losing more than 10 percent of your body weight is associated with a worse prognosis. Even if you start out overweight, don't lose weight. Cancers create hormones that rob you of your appetite and cause weight loss. This creates swelling, worsens anemia, and increases your chance of infections. Use dietary supplement and medications if necessary to keep your weight stable.

18. I didn't want to bother you last weekend. I've been sick for three days now, and I can't walk. Can you help me?

Don't do that. Many conditions can worsen over the long weekend. Patients have developed kidney failure, lost control of their legs, and died of infections because they have waited too long. The emergency room is noisy, slow, and expensive. It can also save your life. Go. If you are very sick, call 911.

19. Can I go on a long car or bus trip?

That depends. What health care have you arranged for where you are going? Will you get out and stretch your legs every hour or two so that you won't develop a blood clot? Are you driving? Is it safe for you to be driving? Are you in too much pain from cancer or surgery to be driving? Will there be others in the car or bus? Are they healthy or will you catch an infection from them?

As you see it's not an easy question. Use your head, and stay safe. Brief local trips are far safer that the 15-day bus trip to the other coast. You may feel intimidated about asking the bus driver to pull over at the local emergency room when you are ill.

20. Does my insurance pay for this?

Usually yes. Most oncology treatments are routinely paid for by insurers. It would be unusual for an oncologist to use treatments that wouldn't be ordinarily paid for. But, at times, off-label or investigational treatments may be denied. You can protect yourself in a number of ways including working carefully with the relevant drug company.

21. Who can help me pay for the expensive cancer pills?

    Lots of resources are available to help. Pharmaceutical companies, foundations, and local support groups are places to start. Alternative treatments should also be considered, such as using IV drugs that may be reimbursed at a much better rate through a different section of your insurance.

22. Why do the cancer drugs cost so much? The drug companies make enough money.

    Complicated question. But they do. Market forces, research expenses, regulatory requirements, and liability worries are some of the big reasons. It isn't going to be easy to change, but public pressure has resulted in major price changes for HIV drugs. More effective cancer advocacy is needed.

23. Is it worth going through all of the pain and suffering of the treatment when I'm just going to die anyway?

    The best answer to this very common but very general question is the following: All of us are going to die, that's understood. And many of us are "ready" to die. Many don't fear death. But most people have a normal and appropriate fear of suffering and wish to avoid it at all costs. Examples abound of types of cancers where treatments greatly relieve suffering. Breast cancer that has spread to the bones is an example of where many easily tolerated treatments are available. They can also prevent years of suffering. Many who ask this question are also suffering from depression, which may need to be treated separately.

24. My grandmother died in the 1970s of her ovarian cancer. She suffered so much from her treatments, why should I treat my breast cancer now?

    Good question. So many advances have been made in the last generation that make treatments more tolerable. There are now much better medications for nausea and vomiting, as well as drugs that can prevent and treat infections. In addition, we now use far better drugs, many of which are more specifically able to target your cancer. Unfortunately, in the past, patients were treated with drugs that were barely tolerable.

25. Am I too old to be treated?

Age has little to do with how well you can tolerate cancer treatments. Far more important is how healthy and functional you are. Can you walk? Are you disabled with COPD (chronic obstructive pulmonary disease). Many elderly people in their seventies, eighties, and nineties have benefited from cancer treatment for years. Don't let ageism set in. If a 75-five-year-old can climb Mount Everest, you might be able to be treated. Keep in shape.

26. Are my children at a higher risk of getting cancer now?

For most cancers, the answer is yes, but the risk is only slightly higher. You might use this increased risk as good motivation to both lower your risk of developing cancer as well as to reduce behaviors and exposures that promote the development of cancer.

27. Which tests should my family get to find their cancers early?

Routine tests that are appropriate for most people include the obvious mammograms, pap smears, colonoscopies, and skin exams. The best plans are to have your family members follow up with a good primary care physician who will be aggressive with their follow-up. Just knowing that there is cancer in the family may help them be more attentive to their habits and health.

28. How could my cancer return if it was all removed?

All visible evidence of your cancer was removed. Microscopic hidden areas of cancer are the reason why so many people have it return. When you hear your surgeon say "I got it all" that only means that he has removed all obvious evidence. For certain types of cancer, you may be offered chemotherapy or radiation treatments to reduce the chance of metastasis. This is important.

29. How could my cancer return if the tests are all normal?

   Even the most sophisticated lab, X-ray and CAT scans tests are unable to detect minute amounts of cancer. Patients are frequently surprised when they have normal tests for years but then, unfortunately, suffer a recurrence. Hopefully with improved biological tests, we will be able to better detect residual cancer.

30. If my blood test is abnormal but my scans are normal, where is my cancer?

   Frequently lab tests are more sensitive and are better able to find cancer than are radiology studies. As the lab become better, this will happen more often. Given enough time, unfortunately, your cancer may show up on your tests. This demonstrates the old adage that early cancer is hard to detect, but easy to treat. Advanced cancer is easy to detect but hard to treat.

31. Are there any other treatment options?

   This is a great question, but it needs to be answered by your oncologist or surgeon after a thorough evaluation. For many cancers, many options now exist. Ask about those for organ preservation as well as ones that limit long-term side effects. Remember, you need to be fully aware of the treatment options and side effects. Both chemotherapy and radiation therapy can have long-term side effects.

32. Will this herbal supplement affect my treatments?

   Don't know. Nobody does. Not even the company that makes the product. It may help, or it may hurt. Almost none of these herbal supplements have been tested when used together with your chemotherapy or radiation therapy.

33. I have no energy. What can you do to help?

   Many things can deplete your energy level including your cancer, your treatment, and vitamin and other deficiencies. So can depression, thyroid diseases, low blood pressure, and dehydration. By treating depression, you may help your energy level. Weight loss with cancer is common. As this happens your blood pressure medication dose may be too high for your lower weight. This is another common cause of weakness.

34. Why do I have to see you again? They got it all.

They did? At the operation, they removed all of the cancer that they could see. Far more might remain.

35. I've got cancer, and I'm going to die. Why do I have to quit smoking now?

For many years patients and physicians both had the same attitude. If all is lost and you enjoy smoking, don't stop now. Well, all will be lost if you continue to smoke. Rarely are smokers lucky enough to respond to cancer treatment. Smokers also have more complications.

36. Can I have my cataracts or knees operated on?

Many people have a list of operations and procedures that they have been waiting to finish. When the need for cancer care arrives, anything sounds better, even cataracts or a knee operation or dental surgery. You and your oncologist need to set priorities and decide what treatment or procedure is most important.

37. Why do I need to have my teeth taken care of?

Proper dental hygiene is critical to your care. It can help to prevent infections in your throat, lungs, and central lines. Dental care is easily overlooked, but very important.

38. Nobody else can run my shop or farm or business. Can this wait?

Your cancer will grow and progress at its own rate. It doesn't know whether you have a business to run or a book to write. Redundancy in your personal responsibilities is always a good idea. Poor planning doesn't mean that your cancer will clear magically.

39. I've lost ten pounds in the last year. Isn't that great?

    No, it isn't. As we said before, any weight loss in a cancer patient is bad. While you may have been trying to lose weight before, this is not a healthy weight loss. By treating your cancer and by good nutrition, you should try to return to your normal weight.

40. I'm tired, I hurt, and I just had an operation. Why can't I just lie here? Do I have to walk?

    Everyone can see that you are uncomfortable, but sometimes you just have to push yourself.

41. I haven't had a bowel movement in four days. Why does my belly hurt?

    It probably hurts from constipation. Many times patients will believe that since they haven't been eating too well, they don't have to move their bowels every day. After several days without a BM, you become nauseated and start to have abdominal pain. Pain, nausea medications, and inactivity all contribute to constipation, which in turn leads to abdominal pain, bloating, and nausea.

42. What side effects from treatment am I most likely to get?

    Fatigue, nausea, constipation, and occasional vomiting all can occur. With proper medications and preparation, you should be able to limit the amount of nausea and vomiting as well as treat the constipation. Fatigue is harder to overcome.

43. When am I done with chemotherapy?

    That depends on the type of cancer, the goals of your therapy, and your lab tests and scans that monitor your treatments. If you are receiving adjuvant treatment to help reduce the chance of recurrence, there is usually a defined period of time for which you will be treated. If your cancer has spread, you may be treated until either a complete remission is obtained or until your cancer progresses.

44. Can I go on a long trip to a family reunion?

    If you are feeling well and think that you are strong enough to be able to make the event, then go and have fun. Be safe and make sure to bring enough of your medications. If, on the other hand, you are ill, feel weak, or are in pain, maybe the event could come to you.

45. Should I go on a study?

After careful deliberation, it might be a good idea. You and your oncologist need to carefully and objectively consider whether or not it's in your best interest. Many studies allow you access to the latest therapies; others, however, may be outdated or poorly thought out.

46. What about this latest new advance in the newspaper?

We're all glad that there are many new advances reported almost daily. Translating them into therapies that are appropriate for you in the community oncology clinic may take years. Series of other clinical trials may need to be done for the treatment to become standard. More studies need to occur for the treatment to gain regulatory approval from Medicare, Medicaid, and others.

47. Whom do I call if I get sick at night or on a weekend?

Don't delay till next week if you are ill. Many cancer related complications can worsen within several hours. Spinal cord compression, dehydration, kidney failure, infections, and sepsis are all common cancer-related problems that can't wait. If in doubt, get it checked out.

48. If I don't lose my hair is the treatment not working?

Most cancer treatments don't cause hair loss. Only a few do, but the visual and cosmetic effect is dramatic. Many newer creative prostheses are available that help overcome the hair loss. When your hair returns, it is often softer and finer. It may also be curly. A real chemotherapy "permanent."

49. Can I delay my treatment for a family event or trip?

Delaying your treatment may or may not make a big difference to your cancer prognosis. That depends on the reason for it and the length of the trip. It also depends on the status of your cancer. If you have recently been diagnosed with an advanced cancer, generally it is a better idea to have it treated first and travel later. On the other hand, if your cancer has been removed or is in remission, then travel may be appropriate.

50.   Am I disabled?

This is a good question. But that depends on the status of your cancer, the treatment that you will need, and what you're physically able to do. For private disability claims, your primary care physician or oncologist can often fill out forms and make a determination. But for Medicare disability, usually those determinations are made by the Federal offices themselves. While you should carefully consider your disability rights, also consider that for your self-esteem and sense of self-worth, you might want to continue, even if part time, in your work.

Resources

WEB SITES

The number of Web sites and organizations available on the Internet to the patient can be overwhelming. I have deliberately been very selective in listing a limited number of sites.

The most trustworthy sites for patients are:

CANCER.NET
http://www.cancer.net/portal/site/patient

This site is run by ASCO, the American Society of Clinical Oncologists, an organization made up of practicing medical, radiation, and surgical oncologists. I and many other practicing oncologists belong to this organization. The site closely adheres to recommendations based on clinical research.

CANCER.GOV
http://www.cancer.gov/

This National Cancer Institute (NCI) sponsored site is also comprehensive and scientifically based. This resource can be used to search thousands of active clinical trials, as well. The NCI sponsors studies throughout the country and at the main NIH in Bethesda, Maryland. The NCI also sponsors training programs for physicians. My oncology training was at the NCI in Bethesda.

NCCN
http://www.nccn.org/

The National Comprehensive Cancer Network is a not-for-profit organization made up of more than 20 very large cancer centers. World experts on almost any cancer can be found at these institutions. The NCCN has been at the forefront of the effort to standardize treatment guidelines for most cancers. The physician oriented guidelines are available on the website now. The patient oriented guidelines are to be available soon according to their website.

ACCC
http://accc-cancer.org/
http://accc-cancer.org/cancer_care/patients/

This organization of community cancer centers has been in existence since 1974. It is made up of all types of oncologists (medical, radiation, and surgical), as well as administrators, pharmacists, and executives. In addition to helping oncology programs, it helps with reimbursement and serves as an advocate on government and legislative issues.

Its Web site includes a great listing of resources. Patient-centered resources include patient advocacy groups, drug reimbursement hotlines, financial and travel assistance, and a listing of clinical trials. You may find these easiest through the site map. The listing of patient advocacy groups in particular is concise, comprehensive, easy to use. and lists major reputable organizations.

ACS
http://www.cancer.org/docroot/home/index.asp

The American Cancer Society participates in prevention, advocacy, research, educational, and service activities. Its Web site includes helpful resources, such as a bookstore, statistical facts, clinical trial information,

information on smoking, and other support information. There is a section to also record patient stories.

ONS ONCOLOGY NURSING SOCIETY
http://www.ons.org/

This is a professional oncology organization run by nurses. It helps oncology nurses with resources in the areas of patient care, research, administration, and education. It has a useful patient education section to its Web site that includes a section on cancer symptoms.

MEDICARE
http://www.medicare.gov/

This is the official Web site for the government Medicare program. It has been improved and has recently become more user friendly. It has been updated to include information on Medicare prescription drug plans, known as 'Medicare D' plans.

SOCIAL SECURITY DISABILITY
http://www.ssa.gov/disability/

This Web site provides a starting point for finding out about applying for social security disability. You will need to apply in person at your local social security office.

FOUNDATIONS

This is a partial listing of foundations and funds that provide financial support for patients. Some of them only apply to certain types of cancers or to specific drugs. You should try to obtain help even if you worry that you may not be eligible. Many of them are very charitable and often provide assistance to those whose income is several times higher than the federal poverty level.

Patient Advocate Foundation (PAF)
700 Thimble Shoals Boulevard.
Newport News, VA 23606
866-512-3861

Patient Access Network (PAN)
PO Box 221858
Charlotte, NC 28222-1858
888-316-7263
www.patientaccessnetwork.org

Chronic Disease Fund (CDF)
10880 John W. Elliott Drive, Suite 400.
Frisco, TX 75034
877-968-7233
www.cdfund.org

Cancer Care
275 Seventh Avenue, 22nd Floor
New York, NY 10001
800-813-4673
www.cancercare.org

Novartis Patient Assistance Program
PO Box 66556
St. Louis, MO 63166-6556
800-277-2254

Healthwell Foundation
PO Box 4133
Gaithersburg, MD 20885-4133
800-675-8416
www.healthwellfoundation.org

Needy Meds
120 Western Avenue
Gloucester, MA 01930
www.needymeds.com

AZ & Me (Astra Zeneca)
PO Box 66551
St. Louis, MO 61366-6551
800-292-6363
www.azandme.com

FirstRESOURCE
Pfizer Inc., 1st Resource
PO Box 339
San Bruno, CA 94066-0339
877-744-5675
www.pfizeroncology.com

Bristol Meyers Squib Patient Assistance Foundation
PO Box 1058
Somerville, NJ 08876
800-736-0003
www.bmspaf.com

Glasko Smith Kline-Access
PO Box 52046
Phoenix, AZ 85072-2046
866-518-4357
www.gsk-access.com

Lilly Medicare Answers
PO Box 66977
St. Louis, MO 63166-6977
877-795-4559
www.lillymedicareanswers.com

National Organization of Rare Disorders (NORD)
55 Kenosia Avenue
PO Box 1968
Danbury, CT 06813
866-924-0100
www.rarediseases.org

Schering Plough
C/O Accessmed
6900 College Boulevard, Ste. 1000
Overland Park, KS 66211
800-521-7157
www.schering-plough.com

RX Hope
PO Box 5836
Somerset, NJ 08875
1-732-507-7400
www.RXHope.com

Nexavar Reach Program
PO Box 220765
Charlotte, NC 28222-0765
1-866-639-2827
www.nexavar.com

Patient Services Inc.
PO Box 1602
Midlothian, VA 23113
1-800-366-7741
www.uneedpsi.org

Bridges to Access
PO Box 29038
Phoenix, AZ 85038-9038
1-866-728-4368
www.bridgestoaccess.com

Commitment to Access
PO Box 29038
Phoenix, AZ 85038-9038
1-866-265-6491
www.commitmenttoaccess.gsk.com

HIGH-RISK POOLS

Numerous states have created high-risk insurance pools. Use the information available through the phone numbers below to see if you could be eligible. These programs can be incredible useful if you unfortunately find yourself uninsured and ill.

NASCHIP*

The National Association of State Comprehensive Health Insurance Plans (NASCHIP) http://www.naschip.org/

This organizations website lists information on state high risk insurance pools. These insurance pools serve people who are uninsurable for medical reasons.

> Alabama (for portability only)
> *Alabama Health Insurance Plan*
> Phone (866) 467-8725 or (907) 269-7900
>
> Alaska
> *Alaska Comprehensive Health Insurance Association*
> Phone (402) 501-8701
>
> Arkansas
> *Arkansas Comprehensive Health Insurance Pool*
> Phone (800) 285-6477 or (501) 370-4234
>
> California
> *California Major Risk Medical Insurance Program*
> Phone (916) 324-4695 or (800) 289-6574
>
> Colorado
> *CoverColorado*
> Phone (303) 863-1960

---

*This information is printed with permission from NASCHIP.

Connecticut
Connecticut Health Reinsurance Association
Phone (800) 842-0004

Florida (not open for new enrollees)
Phone (850) 309-1200

Georgia
Phone (800) 656-2298 or (404) 656-2070

Idaho
Idaho Individual High Risk Reinsurance Pool

Illinois
Illinois Comprehensive Health Insurance Plan
Phone (800) 367-6410 or (217) 782-6333

Indiana
Indiana Comprehensive Health Association
Phone (317) 614-2000

Iowa
Iowa Comprehensive Health Association
Phone (866) 590-6662 or (402) 397-7300

Kansas
Kansas Health Insurance Association
Phone (800) 362-9290 or (785) 296-7850

Kentucky
Kentucky Access
Phone (866) 405-6145 or (502) 573-1026

Louisiana
Louisiana Health Insurance Association
Phone (800) 736-0947 or (225) 926-6245

Maryland
Maryland Health Insurance Plan
Phone (888) 444-9016 or (410) 576-2055

Minnesota
Minnesota Comprehensive Health Association
Phone (952) 593-9609

Mississippi
Mississippi Comprehensive Health Insurance Risk Pool
Phone (888) 820-9400 or (601) 899-9967

Missouri
Missouri Health Insurance Pool
Phone (816) 531-6405 ext. 101 or (800) 821-2231

Montana
Montana Comprehensive Health Insurance Association
Phone (406) 437-5261 or (800) 447-7228 ext. 3474

Nebraska
Nebraska Comprehensive Health Association
Phone (402) 548-4593

New Hampshire
New Hampshire Health Plan
Phone (603) 225-6633

New Mexico
New Mexico Medical Insurance Pool
Phone (505) 622-4788 or (505) 424-7105

North Carolina
North Carolina Health Insurance Risk Pool
Phone (919) 783-5766

North Dakota
Comprehensive Health Association of North Dakota
Phone (800) 737-0016 or (701) 282-1235

Ohio
Phone (614) 644-2658

Oklahoma
Oklahoma Health Insurance High Risk Pool
Phone (405) 741-8434 or (877) 793-6477

Oregon
Oregon Medical Insurance Pool
Phone (503) 373-1692

Pennsylvania
Phone (717) 787-2317

South Carolina
South Carolina Health Insurance Pool
Phone (800) 868-2500 ext. 42757 or (803) 788-0500 ext. 42757

South Dakota
South Dakota Risk Pool
Phone (605) 773-3148

Tennessee
TennCare Program
Contact Tennessee area county medical assistance offices, or
Phone (615) 253-8576

Texas
Texas Health Insurance Risk Pool
Phone (888) 398-3927

Utah
Utah Comprehensive Health Insurance Pool
Phone (801) 333-5392 or (801) 485-2830

Vermont
Phone (802) 828-2900

Washington
Washington State Health Insurance Pool
Phone (800) 877-5187 or (360) 766-6336

West Virginia
AccessWV
Phone (304) 558-6279 etx. 1175

Wisconsin
Wisconsin Health Insurance Risk Sharing Plan
Phone (608) 441-5777

Wyoming
Wyoming Health Insurance Pool
Phone (307) 777-7401

Index

Abraxane, breast cancer, 164
Acceptance, illness, 10, 15, 39
    cancer diagnosis, 11–13
    grief cycle and, 120
Acute myeloid leukemia (AML), 209–210
Adriamycin, 98
Advocacy groups, 233–236
Age
    prostate cancer and, 190
    treatment options and, 82
Ageism, 82
Alemtuzumab. See Campath
Alimta (pemetrexed), 178
Aloxi (palonosetron), 99, 152
Alternative treatment, 4, 40, 227–230
American Society of Clinical Oncology (ASCO), 111
AML. See Acute myeloid leukemia
Anastrozole. See Arimidex
Anger, grief cycle and, 120
Anzemet (dolasetron), 99, 152
Appendix, 243–253

Appointments
    behavior during, 13
    companion brought to, 13, 40, 126–127
    family members attending, 126–127
    first, 13, 18–19
    follow–up, 133
    note taking, 13
    showing up for, 26, 128–129
    tryout, 18–19
    wait time, reasonable, 22
    what to eat/wear, 36–37
Aprepitant. See Emend
Aranesp (darbepoetin), 99
Aredia (pamidronate), 153
Arimidex (anastrozole), 163–164
Aromasin (exemestane), 164
Arthritis, treating, 127–128
Ascites, 185
ASCO. See American Society of Clinical Oncology
Attitude
    depression and, 122
    hands-on practical help and, 237

oncology team, 31
    patient, 1, 7, 14–15, 31–32
Avastin (bevacizumab)
    breast cancer, 164
    colon cancer, 170
    lung cancer, 178
Axitra (fondaparinux), 146
Azacitidine. See Vidaza

Bargaining, grieving process and, 121
Behavior, 7
    appointments and, 13
Bendamustine. See Treanda
Bevacizumab. See Avastin
Bexarotene. See Targretin
Bexxar (tositumomab), 198
Bias
    patient, 10–11
    physician, 10
Bicalutamide. See Casodex
Biofeedback, 130
Blood cancers, 196–211
    leukemia, chronic, 206–210
    lymphoma, 196–202
    myelodysplasia, 202–203
    myeloma, 203–206
Blood clots, 146

265

Blood counts, chemotherapy
  drug influence on,
  101–102
Body language, 19, 59
Bonding
  oncology team, 29–38
  patient-physician
    relationship, 19, 22–23
Bone problems, 153
  breast cancer and, 162
  prostate cancer and, 192
Bortezumib. *See* Velcade
Bowel troubles, 148–149
  ovarian cancer, 187–188
BRACAnalysis, 186
Brain tumors, 157–159
  aggressive, 158
  long-term side effects,
    158–159
  removing, 157
  treatment, 157–158
Breast cancer, 159–164
  bone problems, 162
  chemotherapy, 159–160
  drugs for, 163–164
  early detection, 159
  gene studies, 161
  large, 161–162
  metastatic, 162–163
  rash, 163
  reconstructive surgery
    after, 161
  spread of, 163
  stage I, 160
  surgery, 160–161
Burden of cancer cells, 101

CA 19-9, 189–190
Campath (alemtuzumab),
  207
Camptosar (irinotecan), 171
Cancer. *See also* Sudden
    cancer panic
    syndrome; *specific
    types of cancer*
  advanced, 13
  body sites, 40, 41
  causes, 41
  cells
    dumb (sensitive), 41–42
    growth of, 45
    smart (resistant), 41–42
  curing, 45

detection, 46
diagnosing, accepting,
  11–13
doctor's explanation of, 39
incidence, 43
metastatic, 98, 101–103
mythology, 4
prevalence, 43
primary, multiple, 42
prognosis, 46
smoking-related, 124
spread of
  staging and, 43–44
  time and, 49
  treatment timing and,
    42
stages, 43–44
  determining, 44–45
  system, 2
  treating, 45
  types, 40–45
    care and, 1
    chemotherapy and, 103
  understanding, 39–47
Cancer centers, 48–69
  budget, 59
  care at, 226–227
  choosing, 64–66
  efficiency, 49
  evaluation, 55–57
  experience, 48–49
  geographic areas serviced
    by, 51–53
  goals at, 62
  as last resort, 63–64
  lectures/educational
    opportunities, 55–56
  local oncologist
    coordination with,
    63, 66
  logistical consideration,
    51–53
  long-distance, 51, 63
  physician access at, 61–63
  point of contact at, 49
  records, 65
  relocating to, 51
  selection criteria, 48
  specialists, 58
  treatment advances and, 48
  tumor boards, 58–59
  waiting periods, 49
  what to bring to, 65–66

Cancer research, 107
Capecitabine. *See* Xeloda
Carboplatin, ovarian cancer,
  185
Care
  clinical trials for, 53
  close to home, 60
  continuity of, 20
  decisions, 9
  disjointed, 29
  emergency, 22
  at home, 59–60
  hospice, 212–223
  organization of, 3, 29
  personalizing, 30
  receiving less than
    perfect, 4
  timing in, 32–33
  type of, cancer and, 1
Caregiver Fatigue
  Syndrome, 51
Caregivers, 240–241
  grieving cycle and, 121
Casodex (bicalutamide), 191
Catheters
  flushing, 147
  infections, 146–147
  intravenous, 136–137,
    146–147
  complications of, 146
  port, 136–137
Cetuximab. *See* Erbitux
Check-ups, scheduling
  regular, 129–130
Chemotherapy, 5, 88, 97–98
  adjuvant, 100–101
  administration of, 35–36
  blood counts and, 101–102
  brain tumor, 158
  breast cancer, 159–160
  cancer type and, 103
  CLL, 207
  colon cancer, 170–172
  compassionate availability
    of, 112–113
  diarrhea and, 149
  dose, 97, 99–100
  drugs
    choosing, 103
    combinations of, 98, 201
    side effects, 5
  length of treatment with,
    102

locally targeted, 95
lung cancer, 178
lymphoma, 199–200
metastatic cancer, 98, 101–103
myelodysplasia, 203
myeloma, 205
nausea, 145
neoadjuvant, 161–162
ovarian cancer, 185–186
pancreatic cancer, 189
patient responsibility during, 134
radiation and, 95–96
radiation v., 94–95
side effects, 97
small cell lung cancer, 180, 182–183
smoking and, 123
Chronic lymphocytic leukemia (CLL), 206–208
chemotherapy, 207
DNA abnormalities and, 208
medications, 207
problems associated with, 207
Chronic myelogenous leukemia (CML), 208–209
Clinical trials, 50–57, 234–235
cancer care, 53
cancer center, 48
FDA approval, 54
pharmaceutical company-sponsored, 53, 115
Phase I, 53–54, 55
Phase II, 53–54
Phase III, 53–55
purpose of, 52
selection bias, 50–51
special populations, 53
sponsorship of, 53
treatment, 54–55
schedule, 36
CLL. *See* Chronic lymphocytic leukemia
CML. *See* Chronic myelogenous leukemia

Coding, 73
Collections, 75
Colon cancer, 165–170
chemotherapy, 170–172
detecting, 166–167
medications, 170–171
metastatic, 170–172
spread, 168–169
surgery, 167–168, 171–172
symptoms, 165
treatment options, 169
Colonoscopy, 165–167
Colon polyps, 166–167
Common cancer, pharmaceutical company overemphasis on, 115–116
Common courtesy, 21–22
Communication, 25
explain clearly, 128
oncology team and, 33–34, 128
Community projects, pharmaceutical company funding of, 108–109
Compassion, 24
Compendia, 83
Complaints, 25
Congress, contacting member of, 56, 233–236
Constipation, 148
Cooperative group studies, 48
federally funded, 53
Coping, 144
Corporate oncology, pharmaceutical companies and, 117
Cyclophosphamide, 98
CLL, 207
drugs combined with, 201

Dacogen (decitabine), 203
Dalteparin. *See* Fragmen
Darbepoetin. *See* Aranesp
Dasatinib. *See* Sprycel
Death, 45–47
Decitabine. *See* Dacogen
Deep vein thrombosis (DVT), 189

Delegating tasks, 57
Denial, 12
grief cycle and, 120
illness, 39
Denileukin diftitox. *See* Ontak
Dental problems, treating, 127–128
Depression, 14, 57
grief cycle and, 122
treatment for, 122–123
Diabetes, 131
nausea and, 151
Diarrhea, 149
controlling, 138
infection causing, 149
Dietary supplements, 130–132
Dietician, 56, 130–131
Disability
benefits, 56
brain tumors and, 158
coverage, 86
eligibility, 83–84
Medicaid, 83–84
social workers and, 38
Disease
communicable, exposure to, 139
treating, 127–128
DNA abnormalities, CLL and, 207–208
DNR. *See* Do Not Resuscitate
Docetaxel. *See* Taxotere
Dolasetron. *See* Anzemet
Do Not Resuscitate (DNR), 220
Doxil (Doxorubicin liposome injection), 205
Doxorubicin, 98. *See also* Doxil
breast cancer, 164
drugs combined with, 201
ovarian cancer, 185
DVT. *See* Deep vein thrombosis

Early detection, 13
breast cancer, 159
Edema (swelling), 150–151
Education
cancer center, 55–56

Education (*continued*)
  pharmaceutical company
    funded, 106–109
  treatment, 30–31
Electronic media records
  (EMR), 34
  flaw of, 34–35
Ellence (epirubicin), 164
Eloxatin (oxaliplatin), 171
Emend (aprepitant), 99, 152
Emergency care, 22–23
  evaluation, 129
  insurance and, 84
EMR. *See* Electronic media
  records
Epirubicin. *See* Ellence
Epoetin. *See* Procrit
Erbitux (cetuximab)
  colon cancer, 171
  head and neck cancer, 174
Erlotinib. *See* Tarceva
Etoposide, small cell lung
  cancer, 182
Everyday life, resuming,
  134–144
  hydration and, 137–138
  intimacy and sex in,
    140–144
  travel and, 138–140
  work and, 134–138
Evista (raloxifene), 164
Examination, 128–129
Exclusion criteria, 50–51
Exemestane. *See* Aromasin
Exercise, 132–133
  bone problems and, 153
  edema and, 151

Face-to-face consultations, 91
Family members
  attending appointments,
    126–127
  oncologist relationship
    with, 127
  smoking, quitting and,
    124–125
Fareston (toremifene), 164
Faslodex (fulvestrant), 164
FDA
  drug approval, 6
    clinical trials for, 54
  pharmaceutical
    companies and, 116

pharmaceutical industry
  and, 106
Federal policy problems,
  230–233
Federal programs, 226
Femara (letrozole), 164
Fertility/infertility, 142
Filgrastim. *See* Neupogen
Finances, 37–38, 238
  medical bills and, 74
  pharmaceutical company
    compassionate
    availability of
    chemotherapy and,
    113
Financial help, 56
Flow cytometry, 200
Fludara (fludarabine), 207
Fludarabine. *See* Fludara
Fluorouracil
  breast cancer, 164
  colon cancer, 171
Focusing on yourself, 130
Follow-up care
  home, 59
  oncologist visits, 133
  surgery, 91–92
Fondaparinux. *See* Axitra
Fragmen (dalteparin), 146
Fulvestrant. *See* Faslodex

Gemcitabine. *See* Gemzar
Gemzar (gemcitabine), 5
  breast cancer, 164
  lung cancer, 178
  ovarian cancer, 185
  pancreatic cancer, 190
  side effects, 98–99
Generic drugs, 78–79
Gleason Score, 194–195
Gleevec (imatinib), 208
Goserelin. *See* Zoladex
Granisetron. *See* Kytril
Grieving process, 61,
  120–123
  acceptance in, 120
  anger in, 120–121
  bargaining in, 121
  denial in, 120
  depression in, 122

Head and neck cancers,
  173–174

Health care system agendas,
  17
Health records, personal, 57
Helping others, 238–239
Herbal therapy, 228
Herceptin (trastuzumab),
  164
Histrelin. *See* Vantas
Hodgkin's lymphoma, 197
Home care, 59–60
Home health care, 213
Honesty, 3, 128
  patient-physician
    relationship and, 16
Hormone treatment, prostate
  cancer, 191–193
Hospice, 212–223
  considering, 215–216
  decision, 222–223
  experience, 218–219
  at home, 214
  house, 214
  marketing, 220–222
  questions regarding, 216
  what is, 213
Hycamtin (topotecan)
  ovarian cancer, 186
  small cell lung cancer,
    182
Hydration
  adequate, signs of, 138
  post-treatment, 137–138
Hygiene, 132

Ibritumomab tiuxetan. *See*
  Zevalin
Ileus, 148
Imatinib. *See* Gleevec
Inclusion criteria, 50–51
Innohep (tinzaparin), 146
Insurance, 70–87
  agendas, 17
  basics, 71–72
  coding, 73
  commercial, 77
  coverage, 71
    cost of, 76
    telephone consultations
      and, 94
  employer-sponsored,
    72–73
  high-risk, 85
  information, 65

off-label treatment, 76
outside consultants, 78
patients shortchanged by,
225–226
payment denials, 75–78
Pharmaceutical
companies and,
113–114
policy, 73
preapproval, 77–78
prescription coverage,
78–79
private, 76
Medicare v., 82
problems, 76–78
specialty pharmacies,
79–80
supplemental policy, 81
system, 70
unemployment and, 73–74
Intimacy and sex, 140–144
questions regarding, 141
surgery and, 142
Irinotecan. *See* Camptosar
Iron, 131, 149–150
Ixabepilone. *See* Ixempra
Ixempra (ixabepilone), 164

Journaling, 57

Kytril (granisetron), 99,152

Laparoscopic surgery, 90,
92–93
Lapatinib. *See* Tykerb
Lazy bowel, 148
Legal issues
physician proximity and,
125–126
state, 17
Lenalidomide. *See* Revlamid
Letrozole. *See* Femara
Leukemia, 196–197
acute, 209–210
chronic, 206–210
CLL, 206–208
CML, 208–209
Leukine (sargramostim), 99
Liability
oncologist's fear of, 18
treatment options and,
17–18
Listening, active, 24–25

Long-term care, 86
Lovenox (tinzaparin), 146
Lumpectomy, breast cancer,
160–161
Lung cancer, 175–178
advanced, 175–176
chemotherapy, 178
diagnosis, 175
radiation, 178
small cell, 179–183
symptoms, 175
treatment, 175, 177
Lymphoma, 196–202
chemotherapy, 199–200
complications, 200–201
diagnosing, 200
indolent, 197–198
intermediate grade, 200
medications, 200
symptoms, 199
types, 197

Magnesium, 131, 149–150
Mastectomy, breast cancer,
160–161
Medicaid, 80–84
disability benefits, 83–84
as only coverage, 85
social workers and, 38
Medical bills
collections, 75
discounts, 74
paying, 74–75
understanding, 74
Medicare, 80–84
ageism and, 82
insurance, private v., 82
off-label treatment, 80
as only coverage, 85
Part A, 80
Part B, 80
Part D, 81–82
payments, 83
social workers and, 38
state coverage in, 83
supplemental, 81, 82
treatment and, 71
tryouts, doctor and, 19
Medications. *See also*
Pharmaceutical
companies; *specific*
medications
administration of, 112

alternative, 228–229
blood thinning, 146
breast cancer, 163–164
chemotherapy, 5
choosing, 103
combinations of, 98, 201
clinical trials, 50–57
CLL, 207
CML, 208–209
colon cancer, 170–171
costs, 105–106
development, 105–106
diarrhea, 149
different cancers
responding to one,
110
FDA approval, 6
clinical trials for, 54
pharmaceutical
companies and, 116
generic, 78
indication, 110–111
lymphoma, 200
myeloma, 205
nausea and vomiting,
151–152
off-label treatment, 76
ovarian cancer, 185–186
pancreatic cancer, 190
side effects, 4–5
small cell lung cancer, 182
smoking, 124
trials, 6
weight stability and, 131
Megestrol, breast cancer,
164
Melanoma
spread, 183–184
treatment, 184
Mistakes, correcting, 33
Monoclonal antibodies,
197–198
Myelodysplasia, 202–203
Myeloma, 203–206
advanced, 205–206
chemotherapy, 205
diagnosing, 204
medications, 205
multiple, 203–205
radiation treatment, 206

Nausea, 151–153
chemotherapy, 145

Nausea (*continued*)
  drugs controlling, 151–152
  unusual reasons for, 152
Neulasta (pefilgrastim), 99
Neupogen (filgrastim), 99
Nilotinib. *See* Tasigna
Nongeneric drugs, 79
non-Hodgkin's lymphoma, 197
Note taking, 13
Nursing home expenses, 86
Nutrition, 130–132
  bone problems and, 153

Off-label treatment, 76, 114
  waiver for agreeing to pay, 80
"On call" doctors, 20
Oncologist. *See also* Patient-physician relationship
  access to, 17, 20
  ancillary staff, 30
  availability of, 20
  board certified, 21
  bonding and, 22–23
  cancer diagnosis and, 8–9
  compassion, 24
  emergency, 22
  experience of, 20
  family members introduced to, 127
  first visit, 13, 18–19
  follow-up care, 133
  liability of, 18
  local, 60–61, 126
    cancer center coordination with, 63, 66
  "on call," 20
  patient make-up, 22
  physician-recommended, 60
  preferred provider list, 78
  proactive, 18, 61
  traits of, 20–24
  problem-solving skills, 21
  reactive, 18
  recommendations, 156–157
  respectability, 23
  tryout, 18–19
Oncology societies, 111–112, 234
Oncology team
  attitude of, 31

bonding with, 29–38
communication and, 33–34, 128
record keeping by, 34–35
timing, 32–33
treatments administered by, 35–36
Ondansetron. *See* Zofran
Ontak (Denileukin diftitox), 200
Organ preservation
  radiation and, 96
  surgery and, 92
Osteoporosis, 192. *See also* Bone problems
Out-of-network bills, 59
Ovarian cancer, 184–188
  advanced stage, 186–187
  bowel obstruction, 187–188
  chemotherapy, 185–186
  medications, 185–186
  metastatic, 186
  surgery, 185
  symptoms, 184
Oxaliplatin. *See* Eloxatin

Paclitaxel
  breast cancer, 164
  ovarian cancer, 185–186
Palonosetron. *See* Aloxi
Pamidronate. *See* Aredia
Pancreatic cancer, 188–190
  chemotherapy, 189
  diagnosing, 189–190
  medications, 190
  radiation treatment, 189–190
  staging, 188
  surgery, 189
  treatment, 188–189
Panitumumab. *See* Vectibix
Pathology report, 11–12
Patient(s). *See also* Uninsured patients
  argumentative, 31
  attitude, 1, 7, 14–15, 31–32
  bias, 10–11
  complaints, 25
  confrontational, 2
  demanding, 32
  diagnosing, 8
  doctor dismissal of, 31

information solicited by, 9
insurance companies shortchanging, 225–226
investor and, 105–106
litigious, 2, 31
oncologist relationship with, 6, 16–28
  trust and, 9–10
pharmaceutical companies shortchanging, 225
physician relationship with, 2
primary care provider relationship with, 6
proactivity, 46–47
type of, 1
Patient-physician relationship, 6, 16–28
  active listening and, 24–25
  bonding, 19, 22–23
  common courtesy in, 21–22
  compassion and, 24
  honesty and, 16
  multiple physicians and, 17
  myths/reality in, 16–17
  second opinions and, 25–26
  third party influence on, 25
  treatment and, 17–18, 103–104
  trust in, 9–10, 24–28
Payment. *See also* Finances
  advocacy, 113–114
  arrangements, 75
Pegfilgrastim, 99
Pemetrexed. *See* Alimta
Pharmaceutical companies, 5, 105–118
  chemotherapy, compassionate availability of, 112–113
  clinical trials sponsored by, 53, 115
  common cancer overemphasis of, 115–116
  concerns, 115
  contacting, 234

corporate oncology and, 117
educational resources provided by, 106–109
FDA and, 106
 drug approval by, 116
funding supplied by, 108–109
helpfulness of, 106–107
information sharing, 110–111
insurance problems and, 113–114
investors, patients and, 105–106
medication costs and, 105–106
patients shortchanged by, 225
physician-initiated research sponsored by, 114
profit-driven, 116
regulation of, 106
 issues in, 117–118
resources, 106–107
specialty pharmacy reimbursement and, 79–80
university research and, 116
Pharmacies, specialty, 79–80
Phobia, treating, 127–128
Physician experts, 109
Physician-initiated research, 114
Physicians. *See also* Oncologist; Patient-physician relation-ship; Primary care provider
availability, 125–126
bias, 10, 15
cancer center access to, 61–63
cancer explained by, 39
diagnosing, 8
multiple, having, 17
oncologist recommended by, 60
pharmaceutical education, 107–108
proximity to, 125–126

referrals, 108–109
treatment recommended by, 89
Pneumothorax, 146
Positive outlook, 241–242
Potassium, 149–150
Power of attorney, 220
Practical help, hands on, 224–242
 making a difference, 236–241
Prayer, 144
Prednisone, 98
 drugs combined with, 201
Pregnancy, putting off, 142–144
Prescription coverage, 78–79
Primary care provider
 involvement of, 154–155
 patient relationship with, 6
Problem solving skills, 21
Procrit (epoetin), 99
Prostate cancer, 190–195
 age and, 190
 bone problems and, 192
 diagnosing, 191
 Gleason Score, 194–195
 grades, 194–195
 hormone treatment, 191–193
 surgery, 191–192
 untreated, 190
PSA score, 192–193
Psychologists, 57
Public policy advocacy, 224–242

Radiation treatment, 88, 94–97
 administration of, 35–36
 bodily tolerance of, 94
 breast cancer, 161
 chemotherapy and, 95–96
 chemotherapy v., 94–95
 diarrhea and, 149
 distance traveled for, 94
 long-term effects of, 96–97
 lung cancer, 178
 methods, 94
 myeloma, 206
 organ function preservation and, 96

pancreatic cancer, 189–190
 scar tissue left by, 97
 side effects, 95
 small cell lung cancer, 183
 smoking and, 123
Raloxifene. *See* Evista
Reconstructive surgery, 161
Records. *See also* Electronic media records
 cancer center, 65
 oncology team keeping, 34–35
 privacy regulations, 34
 transferring, 34–35
Rectal cancer, 165
 surgery, 172–173
Relaxation methods, 130
Researchers, 109
 agendas, 17
Research trials, 228
Resources, 254–264
Revlamid (lenalidomide)
 myelodysplasia, 203
 myeloma, 205
Rituxan (rituximab)
 CLL, 207
 drugs combined with, 201
 lymphoma, 198
Rituximab. *See* Rituxan

Sargramostim. *See* Leukine
Second opinion, 12, 25–26
 cancer center, 48
Seizures, small cell lung cancer and, 180, 182
Self-employed
 curse of, 129–130
 work environment and, 136
Sex. *See* Intimacy and sex
Shingles, 200–201
Small cell lung cancer, 179–183
 chemotherapy, 180, 182–183
 medications, 182
 radiation treatment, 183
 seizures and, 180, 182
 smoking and, 180–182
 spread, 179

Smoking
  bad effects, 123
  cancer-related to, 124
  medications, 124
  quitting, 123–125
    family and, 124–125
    small cell lung cancer
      and, 182
  small cell lung cancer
    and, 180–182
  treatment and, 123
Social workers, 38
  cancer center, 49
Sprycel (dasatinib), 209
Staging, 43–45
  clinical, 45
  detection and, 46
  incomplete, 93
  pathological, 45
Stress, relationship, 140
Studies, 50–57. *See also*
    Cooperative group
    studies
  exclusion criteria, 50–51
  gene, breast cancer, 161
  inclusion criteria, 50
  selection bias, 50–51
Sudden cancer panic
    syndrome, 8–15
Support
  financial, 37–38
  groups, 69
    pharmaceutical
      company funding of,
      108–109
  hands-on practical help
    and, 238–239
  smoking, quitting and,
    124
Supportive care insights,
    145–155
Surgeons, 90–91
Surgery, 88, 90–94. *See also*
    Reconstructive
    surgery
  brain tumor, 157–158
  breast cancer, 160–161
  colon cancer, 167–168,
    171–172
  complication rate, 91
  diarrhea after, 149
  local hospital, 91

long-term follow-up,
    91–92
  minimally invasive, 92–93
  options, 90–91
  organ preservation and, 92
  ovarian cancer, 185
  pancreatic cancer, 189
  prostate cancer, 191–192
  rectal cancer, 172–173
  sex after, 142
  smoking and, 123
  timing of, 92
  treatments combined
    with, 91
Survival, improving, 119–133
Swelling. *See* Edema
Symptoms
  explaining, 128
  reporting, 27
Systemic treatments, 94–95,
    98

Tarceva (erlotinib)
  lung cancer, 178
  pancreatic cancer, 190
Targretin (bexarotene), 200
Tasigna (nilotinib), 209
Taste sensations, 57, 131
Taxotere (docetaxel), 98
  breast cancer, 164
  head and neck cancer,
    174
  lung cancer, 178
Telephone medicine, 33–34
  cancer center, 49
  insurance coverage and,
    94
  unfortunate news told
    through, 58–59
Tests, periodic, 133
Time/timing, 13
  cancer center waiting, 49
  importance of, 32–33
  surgery, 92
  treatment and, 37
Tinzaparin. *See* Innohep;
    Lovenox
Topotecan. *See* Hycamtin
Toremifene. *See* Fareston
Tositumomab. *See* Bexxar
Transportation, 237–238
Trastuzumab. *See* Herceptin

Traveling
  medical attention needed
    during, 139–140
  planing for, 139
  for radiation treatment, 94
  resuming everyday life
    and, 138–140
Treanda (bendamustine),
    207
Treatment. *See also* Off-
    label treatment;
    specific types of
    treatment
  aggressive, 77, 227–230
  alternative, 4, 40, 227–230
  attitude and, 14
  brain tumors, 157–158
  breast cancer, 159
  cancer centers and
    advancement of, 48
  clinical trials, 50–57, 54–55
  colon cancer, 169
  combining, 88
  computer protocol
    models, 35
  cooperative, 66
  decisions, 222–223
  depression, 122–123
  development, 89
  education regarding, 30–31
  effectiveness, 88
  experience, 145–146
  guidelines, 103–104
  infertility and, 142
  local, 68
  lung cancer, 175, 177
  Medicare patient, 71
  melanoma, 184
  myelodysplasia, 203
  oncology team-
    administered, 35–36
  options, 88–89, 157
    age and, 82
    liability and, 17–18
  pancreatic cancer, 188–189
  patient-physician
    relationship and,
    17–18, 103–104
  physician recommended,
    89
  plan, following, 27
  port and, 136–137

postponed, 51–52
preapproval, 77–78
returning to everyday life
    after, 134
second opinion, 12
side effects, 145
smoking and, 123
timing, 37
    cancer spread and, 42
tolerating, 145–155
treating other diseases
    before, 127–128
Trelstar (triptorelin), 191
Triptorelin. *See* Trelstar
Trust, patient-physician
    relationship and,
    9–10, 16, 24–28
Tumor boards, 58–59, 91
Tykerb (lapatinib), 164

Unemployment, insurance
    and, 73–74, 84–85
Uninsured patients, 70,
    84–85

High-risk insurance for, 85
job changes and, 84–85
payment problems, 71
University research, 116

Vantas (histrelin), 191
VA system, 79
Vectibix (panitumumab), 171
Velcade (bortezumib), 205
Vidaza (azacitidine), 203
Vincristine, 98
    drugs combined with, 201
    toxicity, 201
Vinorelbine, 178
Vitamin B12, 131
Vitamin D, 131–132
    bone problems and, 153
Vomiting, 151–153
    drugs controlling, 151–152
Vorinostat. *See* Zolinza

Web site resources, 56, 157
Weight loss, 130–132
    edema and, 150

Will to live, 14–15
Work
    commuting, 136
    critical personnel, 138
    environments, 135–136
        clean, 136–137
    lifting in, 137
    returning to, 135–138

Xeloda (capecitabine)
    breast cancer, 164
    colon cancer, 171

Zevalin (ibritumomab
    tiuxetan), 198
Zofran (ondansetron), 152
Zoladex (goserelin)
    breast cancer, 164
    prostate cancer, 191
Zoledronic acid. *See*
    Zometa
Zolinza (vorinostat), 200
Zometa (zoledronic acid),
    153, 162

About the Author

Dr. Fesen, MD, FACS, is a member of the Department of Oncology at the Hutchinson Clinic in Hutchinson, Kansas, and a clinical associate professor at the University of Kansas Medical School. He did his undergraduate work at Rutgers University. He later served as a ward clerk at New York Hospital/Cornell Medical Center in New York City, studied molecular pharmacology at Oral Roberts University, returned to Rutgers to attend medical school, and completed his internal medicine training in Providence, Rhode Island, under Dr. Paul Calabresi, one of the founders of the field of oncology.

As a fellow at the National Cancer Institute, Dr. Fesen participated in clinical drug trials, treated servicemen at the Bethesda Naval Hospital where he was a Lieutenant Commander in the Public Health Service and, during the exploding AIDS/HIV epidemic, he used technology learned from studying cancer drugs to investigate targeting the HIV Integrase Enzyme for the treatment of AIDS. His seminal paper in the Proceedings of the National Academy of Science continues to serve as the foundation for all ongoing HIV Integrase work.

His heart, however, was in patient care. As a partner in a multispecialty clinic for fourteen years, he has helped develop the first oncology clinical trials program in Hutchinson, an oncology-certified nursing program, a local tumor board, and the development of an oncology unit at the local hospital. He continues to support the creation of many other services and practices.

Dr. Fesen specializes in treating patients with insurance challenges and aggressively pursues options for patients with complicated and difficult cancers. His work with local primary care providers has allowed many patients to receive much of their day-to-day care in their rural communities, some as small as five hundred people. He lives, with his family, in Hutchinson, Kansas.